Velocity-Based Training

How to Apply Science, Technology, and Data to Maximize Performance

Nunzio Signore

CSCS, NASM, FMS

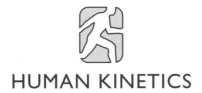

HUMAN KINETICS

Library of Congress Cataloging-in-Publication Data

Names: Signore, Nunzio, 1962- author.
Title: Velocity-based training : how to apply science, technology, and data
  to maximize performance / Nunzio Signore.
Description: Champaign, IL : Human Kinetics Inc., [2022] | Includes
  bibliographical references and index.
Identifiers: LCCN 2020054190 (print) | LCCN 2020054191 (ebook) | ISBN
  9781492599951 (paperback) | ISBN 9781492599968 (epub) | ISBN
  9781492599975 (pdf)
Subjects: LCSH: Athletes--Training of. | Sports--Technological innovations.
  | Speed.
Classification: LCC GV711.5 .S56 2022 (print) | LCC GV711.5 (ebook) | DDC
  613.7/1--dc23
LC record available at https://lccn.loc.gov/2020054190
LC ebook record available at https://lccn.loc.gov/2020054191

ISBN: 978-1-4925-9995-1 (print)

This publication is written and published to provide accurate and authoritative information relevant to the subject matter presented. It is published and sold with the understanding that the author and publisher are not engaged in rendering legal, medical, or other professional services by reason of their authorship or publication of this work. If medical or other expert assistance is required, the services of a competent professional person should be sought.

The web addresses cited in this text were current as of November 2020, unless otherwise noted.

Acquisitions Editor: Michael Mejia; **Developmental Editor:** Laura Pulliam; **Managing Editor:** Miranda K. Baur; **Copyeditor:** Amy Pavelich; **Indexer:** Nan N. Badgett; **Permissions Manager:** Martha Gullo; **Graphic Designer:** Julie L. Denzer; **Cover Designer:** Keri Evans; **Cover Design Specialist:** Susan Rothermel Allen; **Photograph (cover):** Background © Berkah/Getty Images, model © Human Kinetics, Inc.; **Photographs (interior):** Joseph LaTona, LT Visual Media/© Human Kinetics, Inc., unless otherwise noted; **Photo Asset Manager:** Laura Fitch; **Photo Production Specialist:** Amy M. Rose; **Photo Production Manager:** Jason Allen; **Senior Art Manager:** Kelly Hendren; **Illustrations:** © Human Kinetics, Inc.; **Printer:** Versa Press

We thank Rockland Peak Performance in Paramus, New Jersey, for assistance in providing the location for the photo shoot for this book.

Human Kinetics books are available at special discounts for bulk purchase. Special editions or book excerpts can also be created to specification. For details, contact the Special Sales Manager at Human Kinetics.

Printed in the United States of America   10 9 8 7 6 5 4 3 2 1

The paper in this book is certified under a sustainable forestry program.

Human Kinetics
1607 N. Market Street
Champaign, IL 61820
USA

United States and International
Website: US.HumanKinetics.com
Email: info@hkusa.com
Phone: 1-800-747-4457

Canada
Website: Canada.HumanKinetics.com
Email: info@hkcanada.com

E8147

Tell us what you think!
Human Kinetics would love to hear what we can do to improve the customer experience. Use this QR code to take our brief survey.

This book is dedicated to my wife, Tracey, and my daughter, Maia, for putting up with my crazy and constant desire to learn and create, which can render me temporarily unavailable—even when I'm home and many times in the same room. This was no more evident than during the COVID-19 pandemic, when we quarantined for four months in our home in New York.

Contents

Foreword

Nunzio Signore is one of the most passionate, intelligent, and infinitely curious coaches in the strength and conditioning profession. As he proves in this book, he is rapidly becoming a pioneer and one of the "go-to guys" for everything related to velocity-based training (VBT). His work has been an inspiration to us here at the Florida Baseball Ranch, where we train high-level throwing athletes. We have been utilizing VBT for a little over a year, and our results are remarkable. The introduction of VBT to our process has amped up our training's specificity while providing objective, measurable feedback and fresh motivation for our athletes.

When it comes to getting the best return on training time, "specificity" rules. Most coaches and instructors would agree that to get the most bang for your training buck, the activities you choose should be as specific as possible to the performance outcome you desire. Throughout strength training's history, many well-intentioned coaches with incomplete information (myself included) have overused, misinterpreted, and misapplied this concept of specificity. Somewhere along the way, in our pursuit of specific outcomes, solid strength training practices morphed into a load-averse process that became known as "functional training." The original idea may have been sound, but its application watered down the results.

Nunzio Signore understands that while a solid foundation in traditional slow, heavy lifting is vital for any athlete, it doesn't address the temporal dimension of specificity. For high-intensity sports skills that present significant time constraints, traditional strengthening may not be enough to train an athlete to produce force quickly enough to meet the demands of competition. VBT, by providing external feedback on the speed at which we are moving either our body or an object, brings attention to not only the force side of the power equation, but the "velocity" side as well, helping to solve this dilemma.

VBT also takes care of the biotensegral dimension. Muscles don't sit on bones ready to produce power, coordinate and control your movements, or protect inert, non-contractile tissue (such as ligaments, bones, fascia, and joints). They hang off like a sagging rope. Before you can express power, coordinate and control your body, or protect inert tissue, you must remove the slack from the system. In a high-intensity, athletic movement, the best way to remove muscle slack is through isometric co-contraction of all the muscles around a joint or limb. When co-contractions are properly sequenced and synergized throughout the kinetic chain, several benefits are attained: sheer forces are dampened, power is amplified, and connective tissue is protectively wrapped in a blanket of stability. The movement becomes smooth and effortless, and the athlete can accomplish task-related goals while conserving energy and minimizing injury risk.

Before the innovation of VBT, coaches could only estimate time pressure and visually observe co-contraction. VBT, as Nunzio brilliantly explains in this book, provides objective, measurable evidence of time pressure and ultimately training the body to co-contract.

In this text, Nunzio offers a stem to stern look at everything related to VBT and takes the reader on a journey that begins with the theory and history of VBT and culminates in a thorough step-by-step process for applying VBT in programming for all sports throughout an entire yearly plan. Prepare to have your mind opened to an entirely new and incredibly productive way to train athletes. This book is sure to become a staple for strength coaches worldwide and will be a game changer for anyone preparing for a high-intensity athletic endeavor.

Congratulations, Nunzio. Well done.

Randy Sullivan, MPT, CSCS
CEO, Florida Baseball Ranch®

Acknowledgments

Special thanks to Mike Mejia for considering me for this project as well as Laura Pulliam for making me sound a lot smarter than I really am.

This book would not have been possible without all of the great research done on the topic of velocity and power. While there are too many of you to mention here, please know you are in the reference citations and all played a crucial role in the research that went into creating this book.

I would, however, like to give a special thank you to Dr. Bryan Mann, Yuri Verkhoshansky, Tudor Bompa, and the NSCA for much of what I have learned while writing this. I could not have created this text without all of the groundwork you all laid down before me.

A special thanks goes out to my friend and business partner, Bahram Shirazi, as well as Jason Schwartz for his research work on the first few chapters. And lastly, thank you to my entire staff at Rockland Peak Performance (RPP), which many times acted as ground zero in the quest for VBT data over the years—this includes all of the athletes who walk into RPP every day and have the faith in me to help them succeed. An additional thank you goes out to the model athletes—Dante Tobler, Nancy Newell, Josh Loeschorn, and Maia Signore—for providing visual demonstrations during the photo shoot for this text and also to Joe LaTona from LT Visual Media for photographing the shots.

Introduction

Velocity-Based Training: Past, Present, and Future

The concept of velocity-based training (VBT) is nothing new and, in fact, it can be traced as far back as more than 100 years ago, when velocity was about how fast one was moving. More recently, with the work of such pioneers as Carmelo Bosco and Soviets Y.V. Verkhoshansky (*Fundamentals of Special Strength Training in Sport*) and R.A. Roman (*The Training of the Weightlifter*), the athletic-training community has begun to place some visual, or real, numbers and concepts into the equation.

In the 1990s, Louie Simmons brought the Tendo unit to the United States' athletic-training community's attention. The Tendo is a device that hooks to the barbell, plate stack, or athlete and measures velocity in meters per second. If the proper mass of the barbell or the athlete has been entered into the unit, it then provides power output as well as velocity measurements. During this time, Coach Dr. Bryan Mann also helped to further the attention and knowledge on VBT with his excellent work *Developing Explosive Athletes: The Use of Velocity Based Training in Training Athletes*, as well as innumerable published research articles and speaking events at a multitude of seminars on the topic. Through his book and articles, Mann continues to be a driving force in applying VBT to all sport athletes, and, to this day, is one of the premier authorities on research and direct application of VBT to sport.

While I have always been an advocate of pushing the envelope on all things strength and conditioning, I, like everyone else 15 years ago, relied solely on percentages of a 1RM to delegate loads to specific phases of an athlete's program design. This changed drastically a few years ago when I personally began experimenting with VBT in my own facility with my athletes after having read Dr. Mann's book on the subject. I was pleased to find faster results in power, likely because with pinpoint accuracy, I was able to target specific types of strength. I hand-select which of my younger athletes are eligible to use VBT based on their training age, weight room discipline, and ability to exhibit good form. This, in turn, develops my trust for them to efficiently use it.

While I train many high school, college, and professional athletes from all sports, the main clientele in my facility happens to be baseball players. With baseball being such an extremely explosive sport where things happen hard and fast, I have found the carryover to sport to be nothing short of amazing. Pitch velocities and exit velocities have increased exponentially, and gains in sprint times—both in the 30- and 40-yard dash—are apparent across all sports. Simply put, VBT is the perfect fit.

I can tell you this: Since beginning to use VBT with my athletes and getting them to buy in as well, I have found increases in strength, speed, and, ultimately, power (with increases in jump height as high as three to four inches in a single off-season) at a much greater level and frequency. I hope that you find this information valuable and that you, too, can reap the rewards of using VBT with your athletes as I have.

Nunzio Signore

WHAT IS VELOCITY-BASED TRAINING?

Breaking the VBT Code

This chapter introduces the basic concept of VBT as well as why it is a great option for identifying specific adaptations and training zones with your athletes. It also includes a brief discussion on assessing the type of athlete you have in front of you in order to better use velocity to create programs for athletes based not only on the sport but also on the time of year.

WHAT IS VELOCITY-BASED TRAINING?

VBT is a method for evaluating the intensity of a given movement by calculating displacement and time through the monitoring of bar or body speeds. For many years, the standard method coaches used was determining the weight of that load based on a percentage of a one-repetition maximum (1RM). VBT, on the other hand, is based on the speed of a movement or load lifted.

Today's advancements in technology allow us to more precisely focus on the speed at which a bar or an athlete is moving as well as the percentage of loss in velocity from rep to rep or from set to set. The market has propelled the concept and application of VBT in recent years, which has caused the need for more information regarding this emerging technology. That is the purpose for me having written this book. While you don't need to use VBT technology to be a good coach, having a better set of tools will always help a great craftsperson. Don't just use VBT concepts or tools for the sake of relevance; use them to solve problems that are unique to your environment.

Research in Spain revealed a few key findings about some of the benefits of VBT (González-Badillo and Sánchez-Medina 2010):

- People who train with maximal velocity during the concentric phase of a lift or movement attain better strength and power results than those who do not train with maximal intended velocity.
- Velocity decreases fairly linearly across a set of traditional strength training exercises such as bench presses and squats.
- Velocity is closely related to the percentage of the 1RM.

VBT is a method for evaluating the intensity of a given movement by calculating displacement and time through the monitoring of bar or body speeds.

More recently and in growing numbers, coaches and practitioners are using VBT to determine the optimal load independent of 1RM, optimize strength (force), or adjust the load intensity to optimize the velocity and speed at which an athlete can move that load to better produce power as the season draws near (see figure 1.1). VBT is also a powerful tool used to accurately monitor current stress or fatigue on the central nervous system on a daily or weekly basis.

Most sports require approximately 0.150 to 0.220 milliseconds to produce enough force to be considered fast. In more power-based sports such as American football, baseball, or track and field, this time is even faster. While absolute strength, or more specifically, peak force, is still and always will be the foundation for all other types or speeds of strength, the key is to figure out which athletes require more force, or who benefits from working at higher velocities, and the specific loads needed to produce the training adaptations or speed most specific to an athlete's given sport.

Although coaches who implement higher velocity strength work frequently use VBT technology, VBT itself is not limited to developing dynamic strength at higher velocities alone. VBT is an objective method of evaluating intensity of a given movement. So, how exactly is this done? The speed output is typically tracked by a piece of technology or device known as a linear position transducer, which attaches to the bar, or, more recently, wearable accelerometers such as a PUSH Band can be worn around the arm (see figure 1.2), ankle, or waist (the center of mass). These devices help monitor the velocity of a movement, correlating more precisely to an athlete's 1RM. Note that while an athlete's body speed is far more important than simply looking at bar speed during weight training, the key takeaway here is that coaches should look at how using bar speeds in their training can help improve sport speed and the capacity to repeat it.

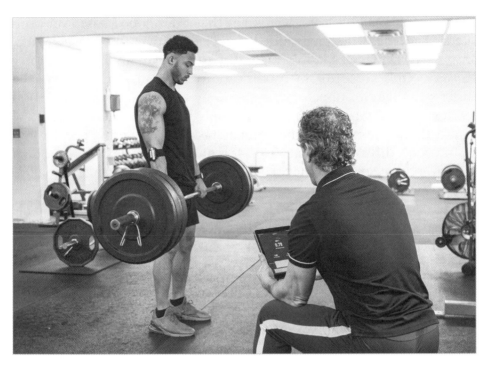

Figure 1.1   More recently and in growing numbers, coaches are using VBT to determine optimal training loads.

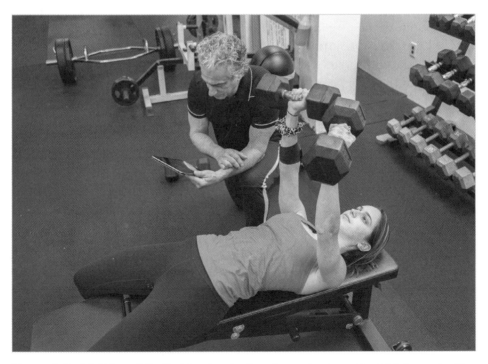

Figure 1.2   VBT is not limited to developing dynamic strength at higher velocities alone. Coaches and athletes should look at how using lower velocities with VBT in their training can help improve levels of absolute strength.

Figure 1.3 is a chart of VBT ranges that I developed based on hundreds of athletes who have trained at my facility over the past few years. Inspired by Dr. Bryan Mann's original chart found in his book *Developing Explosive Athletes* (2016), my modifications take into consideration the different ranges for upper- and lower-body exercises. As you will soon learn, the VBT ranges in figure 1.3 apply to most athletes, but these ranges do not always directly correlate because of varying genetic and training age differences in athletes. It is always best to gather your own data over time; however, I have shared this with many coaches who have reaped amazing results.

The data in figure 1.3 provide coaches and athletes with invaluable external information regarding the speed and intensity of the lift or movement. The data also give instantaneous feedback to lifters about how appropriate the load is for the training session's goal, allowing them to adjust the load or volume accordingly. This can go a long way in helping lifters make better decisions about load intensity when strength is the training focus, or as the season gets near and power becomes the main training objective, finding the appropriate load to use to improve the balance between force and velocity. More importantly, while the percentage-based 1RM has been the standard for many years, it is problematic because it considers neither the intensity nor the daily fluctuations in strength due to stress and fatigue (e.g., lack of sleep, personal issues, the residual effects of a game, the previous day's training session, etc.). These decisions are imperative in order to help create the specific training adaptation we are looking to achieve based on the demands of the sport, a player's position, or the time of the year.

	Rigidity		Power		Elasticity
	Absolute strength	**Accelerative strength**	**Strength-speed (force)**	**Speed-strength (velocity)**	**Starting strength**
	80%-100% 1RM	60%-80% 1RM	40%-60% 1RM	20%-40% 1RM	Bodyweight-20% 1RM
Lower-body speed ranges	<.50 m/s	.50-.75 m/s	.75-1.0 m/s	1.0-1.3 m/s	>1.3 m/s
Upper-body speed ranges	<.40 m/s	.40-.60 m/s	.60-.85 m/s	.85-1.1 m/s	>1.1 m/s

100% 90% 80% 70% 60% 50% 40% 30% 20% 10% 0%

Figure 1.3   Special strength zone ranges and their association to percentage of 1RM.

Reprinted by permission from J.B. Mann, *Developing Explosive Athletes: Use of Velocity-Based Training in Athletes*, 3rd ed. (Muskegon, MI: Ultimate Athlete Concepts, 2016).

WHAT ARE VBT'S GOALS?

This section defines 1RM as well as discusses its relationship to various types of strength. It also explores some of the shortcomings of this standard method, such as residual fatigue from stress and sport, and how VBT may be a much better option when taking these parameters into consideration.

1RM: The Load–Velocity Relationship

A 1RM is the maximum amount of weight that a person can lift for one repetition. This can also be used as an upper limit for determining the desired load of an exercise, as in a percentage of 1RM. This long-standing percentage-based approach has been used to gauge training intensity by helping determine appropriate load percentages to use at the start of a new training program. These percentages range from less than 60 percent maximum to train muscular endurance and hypertrophy to between 90 and 100 percent maximum when improvements in absolute strength are the focus. These percentages also help track improvements at the end of a training block in order to gain insight about a program's validity based on the athlete's pre- and post-1RM testing.

> *A 1RM is the maximum amount of weight that a person can lift for one repetition.*

While traditional 1RMs work, and I have used them for many years, this method becomes somewhat problematic when we consider that strength levels vary before and after a competition or from other stressors, such as lack of sleep or dehydration. These day-to-day fluctuations in strength have been shown to be as large as 18 percent above and below a previously tested 1RM (Flanagan and Jovanovic 2014). For example, table 1.1 demonstrates how an athlete, with a "tested" 225 1RM for the bench press, performed 8 repetitions at 180 pounds (80 percent of his estimated 1RM, or [0.80 m/sec]) on Monday. However, on Wednesday, this athlete performed the same 8 repetitions at 0.50 meters per second with a load of 185 pounds, making this approximately 83 percent of his 1RM and showing a 3 percent fluctuation (improvement) in his baseline 1RM. Once again, on Friday, after a great night's sleep, he hits a personal best of 190 pounds at the same 0.50 meters per second velocity. This is now 85 percent of his tested 1RM—showing a fluctuation (improvement) of 5 percent in his baseline 1RM. But, overdoing it by lifting again on Saturday without adequate rest shows a decline of 8 percent. This downward fluctuation can produce suboptimal results while increasing the risk of injury.

Table 1.1 DAILY FLUCTUATIONS IN PERCENTAGE OF A 1RM

DAY	MONDAY	TUESDAY	WEDNESDAY	THURSDAY	FRIDAY	SATURDAY	SUNDAY
Working load at 80% (.50 m/sec) of estimated 1RM	180 lb	Off	185 lb	Off	190 lb	165 lb	Off
Estimated correlation (%) to 1RM	80%	—	83%	—	85%	72%	—
Daily fluctuation (%)	0%	—	Up 3%	—	Up 5%	Down 8%	—

With VBT, however, we can measure movement velocity as a marker of intensity instead of the traditional 1RM. We can also use VBT to help prevent failure, which as we all know, can be extremely taxing on the central nervous system and equally difficult to recover from. These factors can slow down an athlete's progress considerably. But, let's not get ahead of ourselves—predicting a 1RM with VBT is covered in upcoming chapters.

Using External Cueing

Providing feedback allows people to take that information and make better, more educated decisions. This is especially true when talking about motor learning or the refinement of an athletic skill. External cueing focuses athletes on the effect of their movement through the use of outside information as opposed to internal cueing, where athletes focus only on their body movements or their own inner chatter. Many methods can be considered external cues—a coach's feedback or visual cues from an apparatus, such as a stopwatch or VBT, are two great examples of external cueing.

Research has consistently demonstrated that enhanced motor performance and learning extend across different types of tasks, skill levels, and age groups when using an external focus relative to an internal focus (Wulf 2012). Further studies show that when athletes are given external cueing relative to an internal focus or no focus instructions at all, it not only increases jump height and speed but also enhances neuromuscular coordination (Wulf 2012). Most good coaches and experienced athletes probably already use external cueing when it comes to coaching technique such as, "Extend your hip" or "Drive your feet through the ground" (see figure 1.4). With VBT, we can also get feedback regarding speed or velocity of the movement, whether it is from a bar or the body. Athletes who receive this type of external feedback have

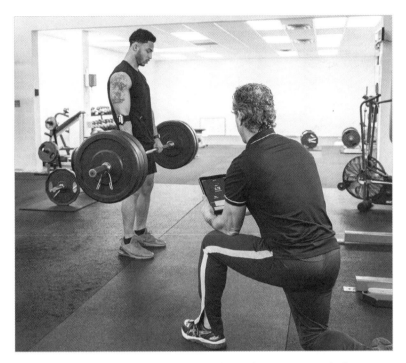

Figure 1.4 While technology-based methods, such as VBT, can help assist coaches, there is no replacement for coaching. Here, an athlete receives important external cues about form from a coach.

shown improved performance results because they were focused on the intent of the activity. VBT also helps to hold athletes accountable for their performance.

Here is an example of how VBT holds athletes accountable: When VBT provides a speed of a lift or movement, VBT is incapable of knowing who the athlete is, which makes its feedback a completely objective analysis of the athlete's performance. So, let's say an athlete performs a bench press in a strength speed zone (covered more later in the book), and the coach wants the velocity to be between 0.75 and 1.0 meters per second. The VBT unit will tell us if the athlete actually performed to the coach's expectation. Despite the athlete thinking the movement was fast enough, if the athlete moved with lower velocity, the VBT unit would confirm so (see figure 1.5).

VBT also taps into the competitive nature of athletes. When athletes are informed that they have one more chance to make the speed before the load is lowered, I have found that 90 percent of the time the intent of the next set increases substantially. As far as training in groups, competitive nature explodes when using VBT. For example, assume three athletes are

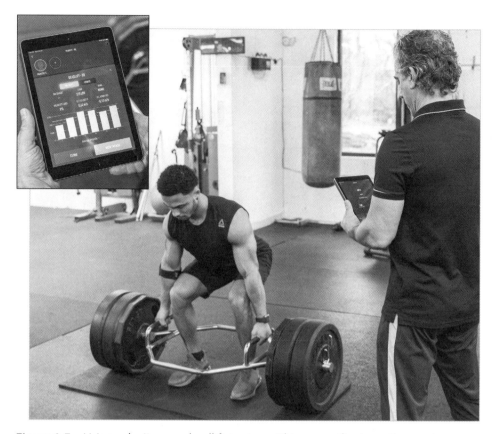

Figure 1.5 Using velocity on a deadlift to stay within a specific strength speed zone.

all working within the same bar speeds. As soon as one athlete moves the weight quicker than another, weight room chatter and the true competitive nature of an athlete emerges. The next thing you know, loads have been increased and concentric velocities have gone up, helping to create these athletes' best workout of the week. To further drive this point home, take a look at table 1.2, where two groups of rugby players were given the same workout with the exact same volume. Results found that the group that received feedback on their work showed greater gains in performance (Randell et al. 2011).

In a nutshell, using VBT for external cueing has provided my athletes with information that enables them to obtain a higher quality of work and volume and thus helps them produce greater gains on the track, court, or field.

Table 1.2 PERFORMANCE INCREASE BASED ON FEEDBACK

OUTCOME MEASURE	FEEDBACK GROUP PERCENTAGE INCREASE	NONFEEDBACK GROUP PERCENTAGE INCREASE
Vertical jump	4.6%	2.8%
Horizontal jump	2.6%	0.5%
10-m sprint	1.3%	0.1%
20-m sprint	0.9%	0.1%
30-m sprint	1.4%	0.4%

Data from A.D. Randell, J.B. Cronin, J.W.L. Keogh, N.D. Gill and M.C. Pedersen, "Effect of Instantaneous Performance Feedback During 6 Weeks of Velocity-Based Resistance Training on Sport-Specific Performance Tests," *Journal of Strength and Conditioning Research* 25, no. 1 (2011): 87-93.

Building Accountability

I must preface this section with this statement: It is my experience and belief that athletes must have a solid base of absolute strength in order to be good candidates to use VBT in their training programs. In working with both youth and professional athletes, I have found that these younger, less mature athletes who do not possess either the adequate strength, nor mobility possibly because of existing growth plate issues, need to focus first and foremost on correct form and gains in hypertrophy. However, as an athlete matures and their training age increases, the athlete generally needs to be pushed harder to actually produce maximum effort concentric movements and continue to create positive adaptations. For such an athlete, VBT can be a game changer. Unfortunately, as with anything, there are no absolutes. Unmotivated or undedicated athletes can cheat the system with VBT. By purposely moving their bar or body slowly during initial testing, athletes can attain lower baseline speeds in order to avoid having to work as hard to match or increase those numbers and metrics later. That is why I require an athlete to earn "the right" prior to allowing them to start using VBT. To summarize, getting immediate feedback on speed makes the intention of the movement clear to hold our athletes accountable.

Monitoring Fatigue

Everything that happens in our lives causes either an action or a reaction. Whether it is training, practice, relationship or family issues, or a lack of sleep, all of these situations can profoundly affect an athlete's central nervous system, or recovery. As previously mentioned, research suggests that 1RM strength can vary by 18 percent in either direction on any given day (Flanagan and Jovanovic 2014), meaning that prescribed percentages can be wildly inappropriate in either direction depending on the amount of stress athletes have applied to their central nervous system.

Autoregulation refers to a system that manages volume to regulate individual differences in an athlete's work capacity based on stress-related fatigue. This can be a powerful tool for a coach helping an athlete to avoid over- or undertraining in terms of the athlete's long-term athletic development (LTAD). Athletes will increase strength by progressing at their own pace based on daily and weekly variations in performance parameters, unlike traditional linear periodization (LP), during which there is a set increase in intensity from week to week. For example, one study showed that the progressive resistance through autoregulation was more effective than the LP model means of programming in increasing the bench press and squat over a period of six weeks (Mann et al. 2010).

By using VBT, we can take these parameters into account by locking into a percentage of a bar or body speed rather than a percentage of 1RM. By receiving a number after each rep on a daily basis, we can see if the weight needs to be decreased due to fatigue that particular day or increased because of new strength gains. For example, assume an athlete has recorded a baseline measurement of 250 pounds (113 kg) for 1RM on a barbell bench press. If this athlete is in a maximal strength phase and the program calls for 5 × 5 at 85 percent 1RM, it would look something like this: 5 × 5 at 212 pounds (96 kg), or 85 percent of 250 pounds (113 kg). We also know that by monitoring this athlete's bar speed with VBT, this particular athlete moves 85 percent of 1RM at 0.48 meters per second. Using this information, let's take a look at table 1.3, which represents three days of the athlete's bench press at a baseline 85 percent of 1RM.

In table 1.3 , day 2 represents what the same day 1 lift might look like after a long week of studying for finals, and a few nights out with friends. When we take into account the various stressors that have been placed on this athlete during the week, according to this athlete's bar speed, the baseline 85 percent now equates to roughly 95 percent of 1RM. Without

Table 1.3 VARIATIONS IN VELOCITY BASED ON DAILY READINESS OR FATIGUE IN THE DEADLIFT

DAY	AMOUNT OF READINESS OR FATIGUE	VOLUME AND INTENSITY
1	Normal readiness	5 × 5 at 212 lb (96 kg): 0.48 m/sec
2	Poor readiness	5 × 5 at 212 lb (96 kg): 0.35m/sec
3	Excellent readiness	5 × 5 at 212 lb (96 kg): 0.52 m/sec

the use of VBT, this athlete may continue to muscle through the next four sets and possibly get hurt. However, getting external cueing from VBT can let this athlete know early to decrease the weight due to poor readiness on this particular day.

Take another look at table 1.3 and focus on day 3. Having aced all the tests and taking better care of one's body, this athlete's next upper-body day shifts to the other side of the curve. Here, the 85 percent that was prescribed now looks more like 75 percent. Removing the negative stressors in this athlete's life (in this case worrying about test scores and nights out on the town) could attribute to the increase in bar speed. It could also be that the athlete simply got stronger. Either way, if the athlete continues to work at this speed and percentage, the athlete may be undertraining and thus not getting the specific adaptation needed for absolute strength.

This is just one example of how getting daily external feedback from VBT not only helps athletes chase the specific adaptation they are looking for but also helps prevent injury or even undertraining resulting from fluctuations in 1RM because of day-to-day stress levels.

VBT allows us to better identify specific strength zones in order to create the specific adaptations we are trying to produce with our athletes. While these velocities are closely correlated at traditional 1RM, there will always be discrepancies among athletes because of genetic makeup and training age. I have personally witnessed the power and competitive environment VBT produces through external cuing when working with my athletes in groups in the weight room.

Understanding the Metrics

Not all velocities are created equal. This chapter discusses the three types of measuring protocols used for implementing VBT. It explains the significance of each and why one metric may be more suitable than another depending on which adaptation—strength, speed, or power—an athlete is looking to improve. This chapter also reviews what eccentric and concentric contractions are, why they are important, and how they play an integral role in VBT.

ECCENTRIC AND CONCENTRIC CONTRACTIONS AND DECELERATION

To understand the different metrics associated with VBT, we must first review eccentric and concentric muscle contractions as well as deceleration in order to know why different methods of tracking velocity should be used. The ability to get in and out of concentric and eccentric muscle contractions quickly and more efficiently allows athletes to better use the stretch shortening cycle (SSC) to produce force at fast rates (discussed in greater depth in chapter 6) and ultimately produce more power. This ability is the gold standard in performance and is a big part of what separates elite athletes from the rest of the athletic field.

During this discussion, keep in mind that VBT only measures the concentric portion of the lift or movement. However, it's vitally important to understand the eccentric portion because it substantially boosts the acceleration of the concentric portion when we monitor bar or body speeds. This makes the eccentric portion of the movement a key performance indicator (KPI) as well when playing sports.

Eccentric Contraction

An eccentric muscle contraction is the motion of an active muscle while it is lengthening under a load. When a muscle contracts eccentrically, it is absorbing energy (as opposed to a concentric contraction which uses energy). The lengthening of the muscle also puts the tendons on slack as shown in figure 2.1.

An eccentric muscle contraction is the motion of an active muscle while it is lengthening under a load.

During this process, a few things happen—the muscle absorbs energy developed by the external load in order to support the weight of the body against gravity, helping absorb shock and reducing the risk of injury. On the performance side, the storage of this elastic energy helps the muscle to recoil in preparation for the following concentric contraction (i.e., acceleration). For example, a countermovement jump improves the eccentric strength of the muscle and helps the athlete store energy more easily in the low position (see figure 2.2a), increasing neural drive and switching quickly to the concentric, or elastic recoil, position, of the jump (see figure 2.2b).

In addition, eccentric contractions require far less motor unit activity (approximately four times less) and consume much less oxygen for a given muscle movement than concentric contractions. These reductions allow an eccentric contraction to handle more force (load), with a lower energy requirement, which may explain why eccentric overload training is essential in the early stages of a strength training program: It enhances tissue prep and makes athletes stronger in low positions. Although VBT is not typically used in this portion of the lift, eccentric overload training maximizes training in later stages when heavier loads are used. It also

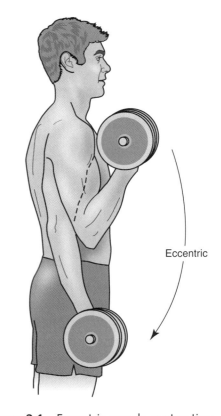

Eccentric

Figure 2.1 Eccentric muscle contraction.

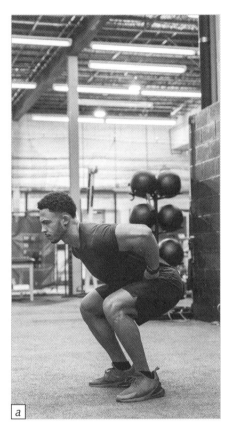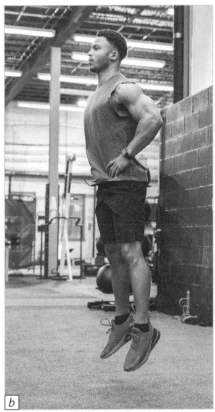

Figure 2.2 *(a)* Eccentric contraction, or the loading portion of a jump, and *(b)* concentric contraction, or the explosive portion of the jump.

helps athletes better absorb and store force eccentrically to achieve a higher end result—to produce a more explosive movement in their sport.

Concentric Contraction

Intention to move a barbell or the body as fast as possible is one of the most important factors for increasing strength and power, and it relies on neural adaptations to achieve this. The increase in neural drive allows the athlete to feel what true explosiveness is all about. It not only requires a great application of force during the concentric portion but also involves selecting the correct exercise to maximize the type of concentric contraction needed (explained in greater detail in chapter 4's section on exercise selection). First, let's briefly focus on what a concentric contraction actually is.

A concentric contraction *uses* energy and will result in acceleration of an object. When a muscle is activated and required to lift a load that is less than the maximum tension it can generate, the muscle begins to shorten. This is referred to as a concentric contraction. Two good examples of concentric contractions are raising the weight during a biceps curl (see figure 2.3a) and coming out of the bottom of a bench press (see figure 2.3b).

> *A concentric contraction uses energy and will result in acceleration of an object.*

However, the speed at which we perform these concentric movements distinguishes whether we are focusing more on strength or power. To increase power, we must train both force (strength) and velocity (the ability to apply this strength). This requires using heavier loads (force) and lighter loads (velocity). During the concentric portion of a movement, the body as a protected device, must reduce the velocity and force of the concentric portion of the rep to guard against jerking the tendons or creating undue stress on the joint when coming to an abrupt stop at the end range of motion. On the other hand, when training the force side of the power equation, there is little deceleration because we are using loads greater than 60 percent of 1RM. Due to the heavier load and slower speed, there is no need for a longer range of deceleration. However, when training with loads less than 60 percent, a larger portion of this concentric portion

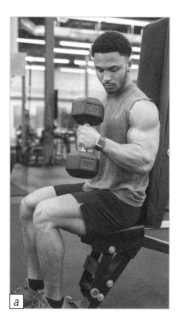

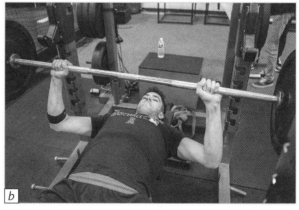

Figure 2.3 *(a)* Concentric contractions during a biceps curl and *(b)* a bench press.

must be used to decelerate the movement in order to protect the body as mentioned. Therefore, to most efficiently train the velocity side of the equation, athletes use ballistic exercises such as jumps and throws. Because the body is being thrown into the air, it does not need to decelerate the load. As a result, higher velocities can be attained because there is no deceleration.

Deceleration

During the concentric contraction, we must both accelerate and decelerate the load. Existing data show that as resistances increase toward 100 percent 1RM, velocity decreases. This act of purposely slowing down the speed of the load or movement is a natural reflex in order to avoid joint, tendon, or muscle injuries—otherwise known as deceleration. Deceleration depends on the intensity of the load we are lifting and the speed at which we are lifting it.

Here is a brief example of how a lighter load requires greater deceleration and vice versa. Lighter loads can involve deceleration of up to 50 percent of the entire concentric contraction. In the bench press, for example, someone using a light load of 40 to 50 percent 1RM could be only pushing during the first half of the exercise while the second half of the movement is spent decelerating. This long deceleration time will have a sizeable impact on the average, or mean, concentric velocity we receive from our training device. On the other hand, loads over 65 to 75 percent 1RM should involve minimal or no deceleration because the load being lifted is not being moved fast enough to affect the average or mean velocity. There are ways to alter the mechanical profile of an exercise such as utilizing bands or chains to decrease the decelerative portion of the lift. For example, when using band resistance, the more stretch the band gets, the more resistance it will offer. This forces the athlete to continue accelerating toward the end of the concentric action in order to overcome that resistance. This, in turn, minimizes deceleration. These higher loads also mean lower velocities, resulting in lower power outputs. Therefore, it is vitally important to use the correct type of exercise and the correct means for measuring the velocity of that exercise. This brings us to the three metrics we use for determining percentages and strength zones as well as which method to use for specific exercises.

Lighter loads can have deceleration of up to 50 percent of the entire concentric contraction.

METRICS FOR MEASURING

Traditionally, resistance exercise intensity has been shown to be the most vital factor in producing adaptations of muscular strength. In recent years, however, another underused factor to consider and measure is movement velocity. When measuring velocities with VBT, we should first be cognizant of what our training focus is. Are we training for strength or power? When distinguishing between strength and power, we must take into consideration both the speed at which the bar or body is being moved in relation to the load and the amount of deceleration involved.

When distinguishing between strength and power, we must take into consideration both the speed at which the bar or body is being moved in relation to the load and the amount of deceleration involved.

One study found that when training for speed or power using loads between 20 and 100 percent 1RM with nonballistic exercises such as your standard bench press or squat, the relative load at which the braking phase (deceleration) no longer existed was 76 percent of 1RM (Sanchez-Medina, Perez, and Gonzalez-Badillo 2010). This tells us that we can get more accurate percentages of a 1RM using loads above 75 percent because there is more deceleration when using lighter loads (remember, the body is being protected as it comes to an abrupt stop at the end range of motion). In summary, when training for strength, using loads greater than 60 percent of 1RM increases the time spent accelerating through a larger range of motion and eliminates much of the deceleration component found when using lighter loads and higher velocities. Knowing which training adaptation to look for will help you choose not only the exercise but also the method of measurement to use, ultimately affecting the accuracy of calculated speeds while using VBT.

Mean Concentric Velocity

Mean concentric velocity (MCV) is simply the average speed during the entire concentric portion of the exercise, including the time spent decelerating through that range of motion. Because strength-based exercises consist of both acceleration and deceleration phases, the mean concentric velocity metric should be used (see figure 2.4). This makes MCV a KPI for training absolute strength exercises such as the squats, deadlifts, and bench presses. It is also the best single velocity measurement to use at the beginning of the off-season when those exercises are performed using loads greater than 60 percent 1RM. For sports where upper-body actions are important and may require more capacity during the second half of the movement, MCV is the way to go.

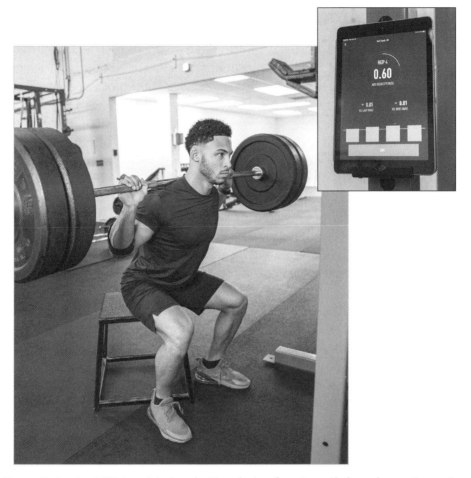

Figure 2.4 An MCV metric is a better choice for strength-based exercises using heavier loads of greater than 60 percent 1RM because they consist of both acceleration and less time spent decelerating (because of the higher load).

Remember that exercise selection matters. While traditional strength exercises (squats, bench presses, deadlifts, pull-ups, etc.) are best for training with medium resistances and higher reps for muscle hypertrophy, or for heavier resistances and lower reps for neural activation adaptations, the slower velocities involved with these exercises do not make them, by themselves, ideal choices for power

Mean concentric velocity (MCV) is simply the average speed during the entire concentric portion of the exercise, including the time spent decelerating through that range of motion.

development. These more explosive power movements can be more accurately measured through the use of peak concentric velocity (PCV), which is discussed next.

Peak Concentric Velocity

A key to continuing to progress and create performance adaptations is increasing the rate of force development, or the speed at which we are applying this newly acquired strength. After a good block(s) of strength (greater than 60 percent 1RM) and dynamic strength (40 to 60 percent 1RM) are attained, higher speeds—depending on what is needed for the sport—can and should be used. This is generally programmed in the final four-to-eight–week block (preseason period) when PCV can be used. This means that the method of measurement will change and the exercise selection will likely change as well.

PCV is simply the peak speed during the concentric portion of the exercise, and it is usually calculated every 5 to 10 milliseconds. This metric is used for ballistic or power-based exercises. Ballistic exercises are movements where force is produced for a very short amount of time before the implement or body is projected into the air. During a large portion of these ballistic movements, the athlete is not actually applying force to the bar, so using an average of the entire movement is less efficient because no deceleration is produced from trying to lock out the rep (see figure 2.5). Exercises such as power cleans, snatches, bench press throws, and jump squats are generally used in this period. Because of the ballistic nature of these exercises, it is important to remember that, although MCV is still usable, it would not be as accurate or efficient, and therefore, PCV may be a better option.

> *PCV is simply the peak speed during the concentric portion of the exercise, and it is usually calculated every 5 to 10 milliseconds.*

Mean Propulsive Velocity

Mean propulsive velocity (MPV) is a bit more involved, but it is a great method for measuring and assessing true muscular power. Unfortunately, MPV is not available on many wearable devices such as linear transducers. Nonetheless, we need to understand the importance of MPV to be able to apply it when devices such as Tendo and GymAware units are available.

While MCV refers to and measures the entire upward portion of a lift (including the braking phase), its accuracy begins to get compromised at or less than 60 percent of 1RM. MPV refers to and measures only the portion of the upward movement during which the measured acceleration is greater than the acceleration related to gravity. In other words, it happens before deceleration occurs.

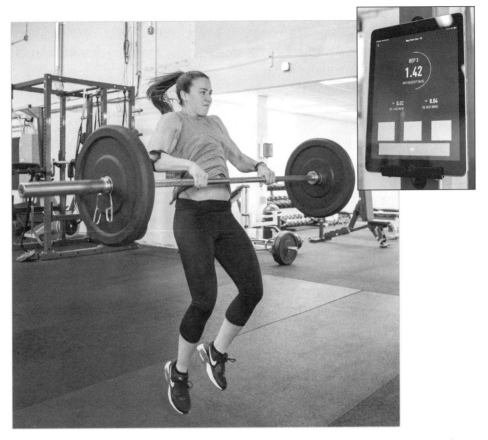

Figure 2.5 Using a PCV metric during ballistic movements, such as the hang clean.

MPV may be a more valid measurement later in the off-season for both traditional exercises when dynamic strength (loads between 40 to 60 percent 1RM are being used, and greater deceleration occurs due to the necessity to brake at the end of the range of motion) and heavier ballistic jumps are performed at or around 40 to 50 percent 1RM when the deceleration is not significant because the upward phase occurs only after the implement has either left the hands or the body has left the ground (i.e., takeoff).

Mean propulsive velocity refers to and measures only the portion of the upward movement during which the measured acceleration is greater than the acceleration related to gravity.

Based on this mechanical principle, the use of MCV related to the entire upward portion of a given movement may be more biased and a less effective means of measurement than the use of MPV with lighter loads. A training system based on MPV may be a better option for measuring performance at both ends of the force–velocity curve, whether it be a jump or maximum dynamic strength ability, such as a 1RM for a back squat.

This information suggests that, by referring the MCVs to the propulsive phase, we can avoid underestimating an athlete's true neuromuscular potential when lifting light and medium loads while training for power simply by taking out the measurement of the deceleration phase. Therefore, many coaches and athletes believe that using MPV in training and testing settings allows for a more effective method of measuring training for strength or power than MCV.

Velocity is a useful parameter to measure during resistance training. However, it is *imperative* to use the correct measuring protocol to factor in the amount of time spent in the deceleration phase of the movement. Mean (average) velocity, especially with resistances more than 60 percent 1RM, correlates well with strength exercises such as squats, deadlifts, and bench presses and can be used when training strength as well as for determining 1RMs. Dynamic strength and power adaptations, on the other hand, typically occur using the same exercise at more moderate resistances (approximately 40 to 60 percent) and require more deceleration. This makes mean propulsive velocities a more efficient method because the decelerated portion of the lift is eliminated when calculating average speeds. Finally, more ballistic types of exercises, such as cleans, snatches, weighted jumps, and throws, are used in training for explosiveness.

Peak power may be a better option to calculate the fastest 5 to 10 meters per second—the closest to in-game speeds—of these lifts or jumps, making them great options during preseason training (see figure 2.6). In a study by Sanchez-Medina et al. (2010), the relative load that maximized mechanical power output was determined using three different parameters: mean concentric velocity and power, mean power of the concentric portion, and peak power. The load at which the braking phase no longer existed was (regardless of the method used) 76.1 percent (+/– 7.4) of 1RM. This is more than likely due to having to apply force for a longer period of time because of the heavier load. Maximum mechanical power output was dependent on the parameter used, making it imperative to select the appropriate parameter according to the type of exercise being done as well as the load being used.

Table 2.1 provides a quick summary of the three main methods of measurement, the various measurements, and the adaptations they calculate.

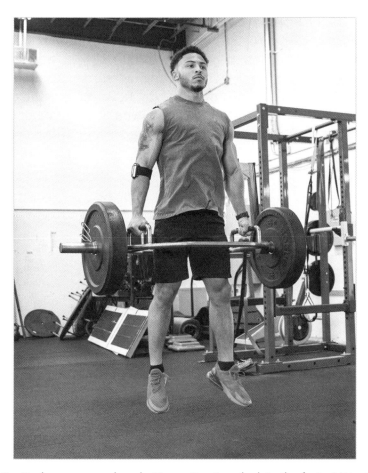

Figure 2.6   Peak power may be a better option to calculate the fastest 5 to 10 meters per second—the closest to in-game speeds—more ballistic types of exercises, like the trap bar jump shown here.

Table 2.1   VELOCITY MEASUREMENT METHODS

METHOD	DESCRIPTION	SAMPLE EXERCISE SELECTION
Mean concentric velocity (MCV)	The average speed during the entire concentric portion of the exercise, including the time spent decelerating	Traditional exercises > 60% 1RM (e.g., back squats, bench presses, deadlifts)
Peak concentric velocity (PCV)	The peak speed during the concentric portion of the exercise, usually calculated every 5 to 10 milliseconds	Ballistic or power-based exercises (e.g., Olympic lifts)
Mean propulsive velocity (MPV)	Measures *only* the portion of the upward movement during which the measured acceleration is greater than the gravity-related acceleration (before deceleration occurs)	Traditional exercises in which dynamic strength loads between 40%-60% 1RM are used (e.g., squats, bench presses, deadlifts)

Hopefully, this chapter has cleared up a few things regarding the eccentric and concentric portions of a movement and the relation of acceleration and deceleration to different percentages of a 1RM. Using the correct metric—MCV, PCV, or MPV—when taking measurements is essential for getting the most accurate readings. We do, however, need to err on the side of caution with using MPV because, even at the time of the printing of this book, the metric is not available at most commercial units, making it an expensive option.

Tools of the Trade

Not long ago, the linear position transducer (LPT) was the only way to measure the velocity of the body or a bar. Now, with the addition of accelerometers, coaches and trainers have various ways to monitor velocity and power output. No matter the tool you choose, all calculate velocity by measuring the rate of change in the body's or bar's position over time. Because each method measures velocity a little differently, it is imperative to perform a velocity profile before you begin training. By doing so, we are using the athlete's specific means of measurement in order to keep data consistent. (Velocity profiling is discussed in upcoming chapters.)

OVERVIEW OF VBT MEASURING TOOLS

Some coaches may prefer one type of measuring tool over another, but the bottom line is each kind measures velocity by a different means. This section discusses what makes these devices different from each other and the pros and cons to consider when choosing the tool that may be most practical for you.

Linear Position Transducers

LPTs such as GymAware or Tendo units are devices capable of measuring displacement in a linear plane (see figure 3.1). An LPT consists of a hardwired measuring cable—otherwise known as a tether, spool, or spring—and a sensor, such as a potentiometer or rotary encoder. The sensor converts the change in distance of the cable to voltage and, ultimately, velocity and acceleration. The LPT also calculates average force using the summed mass of the barbell and the mass of the lifter and

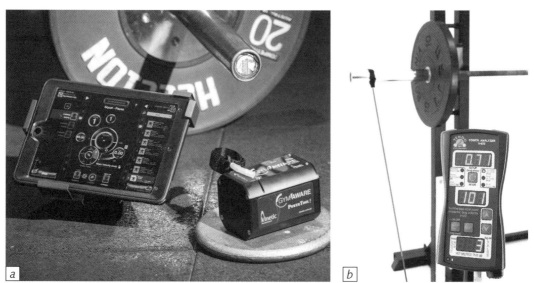

Figure 3.1   *(a)* The GymAware and *(b)* Tendo unit are the two main LPTs.
(a) Courtesy of GymAware; *(b)* Courtesy of Tendo Sport

multiplying by acceleration due to gravity (g = 9.81 m × s – 2). The average power may be calculated for each movement using the average force and average velocity. Using a hardwired cable makes it easy to transition from exercise to exercise without having to restart the device whenever changing angles within the exercise selection. The advantage of using an encoder is simple to see: The data is always a direct measure rather than a calculated estimate.

In an attempt to validate LPT technology, a study was conducted using an LPT that used three jumping conditions (squats, countermovements, and drops) and compared the force plate's values of average force, peak force, and time–peak force to the LPT's values. The study concluded that LPT technology is a useful and accurate tool for measuring movement velocity (Cronin, Hing, and McNair 2004). In another study that also examined the reliability of measurement between the force plate and LPT technology, each subject completed two testing sessions that were separated by one week and included three rebound jump squats with an 88-pound (40 kg) external load. Again, the force plate and the LPT were both found to be reliable in the measurement of peak force (Hansen, Cronin, and Newton 2011).

While the price of Tendo units and GymAware might not be considered as expensive as other measuring equipment, such as force plates, they do present some budgetary concerns for many training facilities, as well as strength and conditioning coaches and personal trainers. Coaches who train athletes either individually, or small in groups, might want to consider different options for their day-to-day monitoring purposes. For this reason, all VBT examples shown will use an accelerometer because it is currently the most practical application used in the United States.

Accelerometers

More recently accelerometers, such as the PUSH Band (see figure 3.2) and Bar Sensei, which are able to accurately calculate velocity, have been making their way into facilities much like mine. Accelerometers differ from LPTs because they use an algorithm to determine where the body or bar is being positioned and when each movement starts and stops. This algorithm adjusts according to the exercise being performed; for example, with jumps, it adjusts through the change in angles when a person moves from a vertical position to a wide position. Accelerometers do not have the hardwired cable to calculate angles; instead, they are preprogrammed to a built-in specific exercise suite. This feature works, but its readings can be slightly more skewed than those of an LPT.

Accelerometers are great for measuring peak velocity (PV), but they are inferior at detecting where they are in time and space. They are usually included in other systems to assist the calculations, but again,

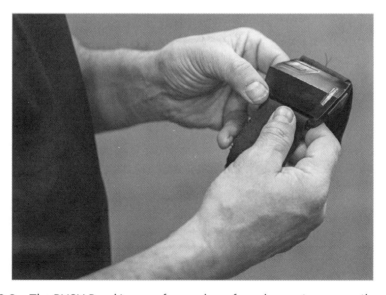

Figure 3.2 The PUSH Band is one of a number of accelerometers currently available on the market.

the algorithms are usually a step behind the technology. Small, subtle idiosyncrasies, such as gripping the barbell and small micromovements, will throw off calculations with accelerometers' algorithms.

Another disadvantage of accelerometers is they currently lack the capability to measure force (in real time) of rep-to-rep sets, which, as we know, is the other half of the power equation. These units only measure velocity. While some companies provide access to force readings via a company portal, there are downsides to this. Users are required to purchase expensive yearly subscriptions, and the readings are not immediate. There are, however, many benefits of using an accelerometer in a group setting. First and foremost is affordability: Accelerometers have a much lower price point than LPTs. Despite being slightly less accurate at pinpointing specific velocities, in a team setting where wider ranges are often used, accelerometers work just fine. Other benefits worth pointing out are that accelerometers are designed to be worn on the body or on the bar, do not require a hardwired cable, can be used anywhere, and require much less space in the weight room. I have about 15 of them in my facility and have been getting great results for years. I do, however, also have one LPT when individual profiles are necessary.

While LPTs and accelerometers both show great accuracy and testing when compared to a 1RM, LPT technology in the Tendo unit and GymAware still seems to be the gold standard and the more valid and reliable way to measure velocity, acceleration, and force variables compared to any accelerometer. However, accelerometers are still a viable option for facilities in the private sector and in team settings where multiple units can be used and a wider velocity range is applied (see table 3.1).

Table 3.1 PROS AND CONS OF LPTS AND ACCELEROMETERS

DEVICE TYPE	PROS	CONS
LPT (e.g., Tendo unit and GymAware)	• Cable attachment makes readings more accurate • Measures force from rep to rep as well as velocity	• Very expensive • Not very portable • Easier to break (cable)
Accelerometer (e.g., PUSH Band and Bar Sensei)	• Inexpensive • Easily portable • Works well in group setting	• Uses a slightly less accurate preprogrammed algorithm • Currently does not read force output from rep to rep

DEVICE SETUP AND DATA INTERPRETATION

This section provides a brief overview of the basic setup for using both an LPT and accelerometer. This is not a how-to instruction manual; it is merely a glimpse of the step-by-step procedure from attaching the devices to reading the information. The setup is slightly different for each device.

As with any device that incorporates the use of data, the best place to begin is by simply starting to use the device. I recommend getting used to the feedback of the unit by reading velocities from rep to rep and seeing if they improve or worsen. Even in these initial stages of learning to use and apply VBT, you will begin to see results.

As discussed in the previous section, many different types of technology on the market are used for measuring VBT. Refer back to table 3.1 for a few of the more popular and most dependable (in my opinion) options for LPTs and accelerometers.

Basic Setup for LPTs

For LTPs, such as the GymAware and Tendo, a thin cable spool attaches to the barbell to measure distance and speed of the bar. The sensors sample not only the rate and distance the cable line is traveling but also the angle. Data can be stored locally on the device or through an online portal in the cloud. The basic setup is as follows:

1. **Set up the device.**

   This step is easy and self-explanatory. Some coaches get concerned with the reliability when bar whip associated with the Olympic lifts causes cable slack. While every unit will have some issues with readings, absolute difference is so low that it should be of little concern. Most of the bar whip comes from very heavy competitive loads, not the typical ones used in sports training.

2. Pair the device to an iPad.

The first step before pairing anything is to ensure that the Wi-Fi is strong and secure. If you train in a basement or an underground weight room, test the saturation of the Wi-Fi connection to each iPad and lock it down.

3. Place the iPad in a convenient and safe location.

For the best functionality, iPads should be placed where athletes can get feedback conveniently but out of the way of weights. Make sure to use a mounting option that allows the tablet to be mobile. Each unit pairs within a specific iPad, but the data are universal, so, technically, any athlete can train off of any iPad or station.

4. Synchronize with the unit's portal through the cloud (optional).

Most of the time, I record data locally (stored on the device); however, there is a great option for collecting data for teams to use. After each iPad is securely connected to Wi-Fi, connect the associated app to the cloud to access a user portal. Connecting is very simple and only requires a username and password. After that, the rest is basically done for you.

5. Set target zones and timers for workflow (optional).

These are great options that only LPTs offer. Refer to the user manual for more information on how set up these functions.

6. Select your exercise.

To get the most accurate readings, all VBT devices come with a library of exercises; however, most research and information refer to the big lifts (squats; d-lifts; and bench and body-weight exercises such as countermovement jumps, push-ups, and pull-ups).

7. Select your load and start your set.

Get into the habit of pushing every rep with maximal voluntary concentric (MVC) action. This just means pushing every single velocity measured rep as hard and as fast as you are physically capable. Doing so ensures readings are as accurate as possible. Slowing down concentric muscle action greatly skews the readings of the velocity measuring technology.

Basic Setup for Accelerometers

LPTs are wonderful, but, as you may recall, they are generally not practical for application in a large-group setting. Because of the high volume of athletes coming in on a daily basis, over the past three years, I have incorporated 14 PUSH Bands for their use in my facility. PUSH Bands are easy to use and a great alternative to LPTs, which take up a lot of space and time in a rack when the gym gets crowded with 20 or more athletes all training at the same time with their own individualized programs. The basic setup instructions for accelerometers are as follows:

1. **Charge the band and download app.**

   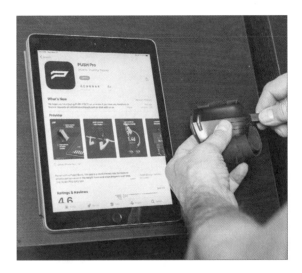

   Most portable accelerometers use a micro USB adapter that can connect to a laptop or a wall connector. After connection, download the app onto the iOS device, launch the app, and click on the menu option to get started.

2. **Pair the band with the iOS device.**

   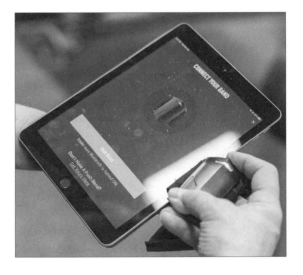

   Every unit has its own way of pairing an iOS device to a band, but all accelerometers currently on the market do it through the use of an app that needs to be downloaded. Note that the band can be connected to only one device at a time, so if the band is solid blue, it means it is already connected to another iOS device.

3. Choose the mode.

While most units come with adapters to enable direct placement on a bar, my experience has seen more variance in readings from set to set when using bar mode due to the possibility of the bar flying out of the hands or off the top of the shoulders when reaching end range.

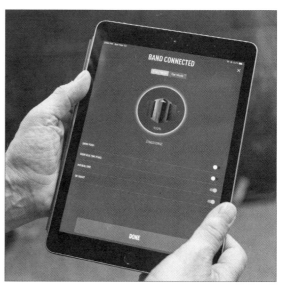

For this reason, I place the unit directly on the body, preferably using a belt around the center of mass exclusively.

4. Place the iPad in a convenient and safe location.

For the best functionality, iPads should be placed where athletes can get feedback conveniently but out of the way of weights. Make sure to use a mounting option that allows the tablet to be mobile. Each unit pairs within a specific iPad, but the data are universal, so, technically, any athlete can train off of any iPad or station.

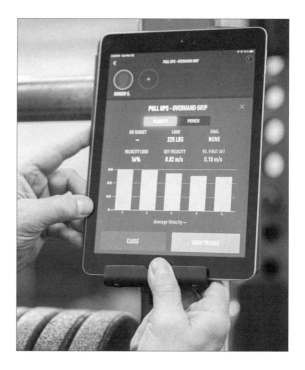

5. Attach the device to a barbell.

Attach the device to the barbell close to the plates so that it is out of the way of the grip.

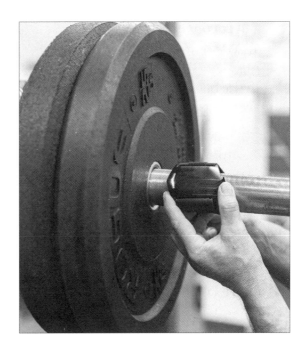

6. Place the band.

Accelerometers can be worn on the arm or the waist depending on the exercise selection. For most exercises, place the band on the upper forearm or the lower biceps (placement is based on the type of exercise being performed). Your mobile app will display the proper band placement for each exercise. Note: For jumps and free movement, most units will include a waist belt that places the band firmly on the center of mass just above the tailbone.

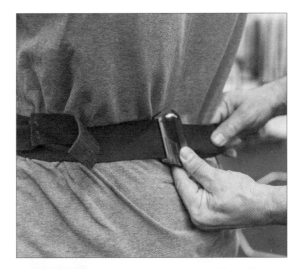

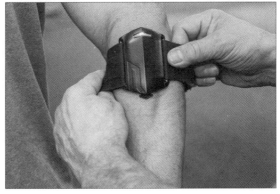

7. Select your exercise.

To get the most accurate readings, all VBT devices come with a library of exercises; however, most research and information refer to the big lifts (squats; d-lifts; and bench and body-weight exercises such as countermovement jumps, push-ups, and pull-ups).

8. Select your load and start your set.

Get into the habit of pushing every rep with maximal voluntary concentric (MVC) action. This just means pushing every single velocity measured rep as hard and as fast as you are physically capable. Doing so ensures readings are as accurate as possible. Slowing down concentric muscle action greatly skews the readings of the velocity measuring technology.

Interpreting the Data

You've gathered the data—now what? Upon completion of the set or rep, we can use the information we have received from the device in many different ways, which, honestly, can be a book within itself. The zones in figure 3.3 are from the same diagram as we saw in figure 1.3 in chapter 1. (Note: For the sake of ease, this figure appears again in other chapters.) Once again, while there are standard speeds that correlate to a particular percentage of a 1RM, it is best practice to create your own zones based on your clientele. These particular zones in figure 3.3 work for my clientele who generally range from 16 to 24 years old.

In other words, the data in figure 3.3 basically say that the heavier a weight gets, the slower it moves. The interesting part about this specific data is that the velocity ranges are labeled by both speed of movement and then the quality that specific velocity zone helps to develop. For example, a powerlifter may stick to 85 percent or more of 1RM for the

	Rigidity				Power				Elasticity	
100%	90%	80%	70%	60%	50%	40%	30%	20%	10%	0%
	Absolute strength		Accelerative strength		Strength-speed (force)		Speed-strength (velocity)		Starting strength	
	80%-100% 1RM		60%-80% 1RM		40%-60% 1RM		20%-40% 1RM		Bodyweight-20% 1RM	
Lower-body speed ranges	<.50 m/s		.50-.75 m/s		.75-1.0 m/s		1.0-1.3 m/s		>1.3 m/s	
Upper-body speed ranges	<.40 m/s		.40-.60 m/s		.60-.85 m/s		.85-1.1 m/s		>1.1 m/s	

Figure 3.3 Special strength zone ranges and their association to percentage of 1RM.

Reprinted by permission from J.B. Mann, *Developing Explosive Athletes: Use of Velocity-Based Training in Athletes*, 3rd ed. (Muskegon, MI: Ultimate Athlete Concepts, 2016).

bulk of training the lifter is developing absolute strength, whereas a football player would benefit more by training within the accelerative strength zone of 70 to 80 percent, allowing the player to get off the line and overpower weaker opponents who mistakenly trained with too heavy of loads in the weight room and failed to capture the same accelerative benefits. But let's not get ahead of ourselves; each of these zones will be discussed in greater detail in later chapters.

Let's suppose an athlete performs a squat with 280 pounds (127 kg) for five reps. Upon completion, the athlete gets an average reading of 0.62 meters per second for the set. According to the data in figure 3.3, this reading would fall into the range of accelerated strength and be equivalent to roughly 70 percent 1RM, giving the athlete an estimated 1RM of 400 pounds (181 kg): $400 \times 0.70 = 280$ ($181 \times 0.70 = 127$). If this athlete's program has prescribed 70 percent 1RM, this reading falls within the correct range. However, if 80 percent 1RM has been prescribed, the number to strive for is closer to 0.50 meters per second, and weight should be added. If 60 percent 1RM were prescribed, then 0.75 meters per second is the target number, and a lighter load is needed.

In a nutshell, VBT allows for both velocity and power data to be given instead of a hard number by using the special zones indicated in figure 3.3. This not only lets us know that we are working in the correct pre-scribed percentage for that day but also helps us autoregulate and take daily fatigue into consideration. Studies published in *The Journal of*

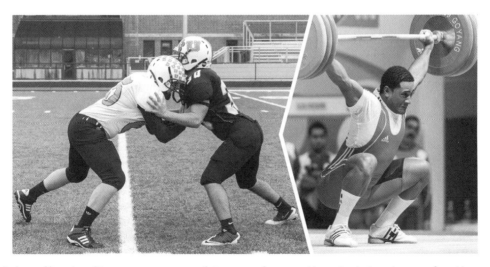

An offensive lineman may need to spend more time training in accelerative strength as compared to a powerlifter who may spend a majority of time training absolute strength.

(a) © Human Kinetics; *(b)* Seung-il Ryu/NurPhoto via Getty Images

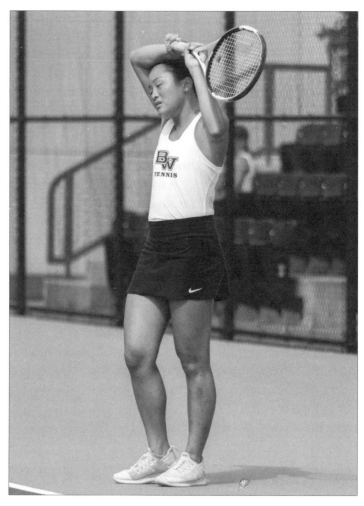

Due to various factors, such as lack of sleep, game play, or overtraining, strength levels can vary by as much as 18 percent, making VBT a valuable method for autoregulating workload.

© Human Kinetics

Australian Strength and Conditioning show how variable strength is from one workout to another. Researchers found that a daily 1RM provided for an 18 percent range of variance. This means that the 75 percent of your 1RM programmed and performed on this day could be anywhere between 75 percent plus or minus 18 percent (57 to 93 percent of your 1RM) on another given day and training session (Pareja-Blanco et al. 2016). This demonstrates one of the most valuable aspects of using VBT—autoregulation and consideration of daily fatigue.

Everyone's needs are different, so a few things should be considered before deciding whether the LPT or accelerometer better suits you or your athletes:

- Is there a need for portability as a group setting?
- Which types of exercises and sports are being trained? Remember, LPTs track angular exercises more accurately because of their hardwired cable. But, if the training exercises are lifts such as squats, bench presses, deadlifts, and Olympic lifts and getting data on force production is not an issue, then either choice will do the job.
- What is your budget and how much can you afford? Price differences between LPTs and accelerometers are drastic, making accelerometers the more affordable option.

PART

II

GETTING STARTED

The Special Strength Zones

The S.A.I.D. principle, which stands for "specific adaptation of imposed demands," states that training should create the adaptation or trait that is needed to excel in our desired sport. However, the type of adaptation needed changes from month to month and from athlete to athlete based on anatomical makeup. One key advantage of VBT is the ability for athletes or coaches to ensure that the desired trait they are trying to achieve is being developed. Every type of strength or trait has a speed. If we are not training in the required zone or at the desired speed, then we are not developing the strength or trait we are chasing. This is where the special strength zones come into play.

In this chapter, we look more closely at these zones and the specific speeds and ranges involved as well as explain what the zones mean, which specific adaptations in performance they help achieve, and the appropriate times of the year they are applied. VBT allows the athlete to pinpoint the specific strength adaptations that fall along the force–velocity curve with greater accuracy. This chapter also covers how to perform a force–velocity profile in the following chapter, but for now, let's get into the special strength zones and how to better use them through VBT.

MONITORING STRENGTH BY SPEED

Every zone is associated with a specific bar and body speed (velocity) and thus produces a different stimulus and corresponding performance adaptations that are exclusive to the zone itself. This better enables us to monitor an athlete's associated velocities and focus on the trait the athlete is trying to develop to help improve performance specific to that athlete's sport (see table 4.1).

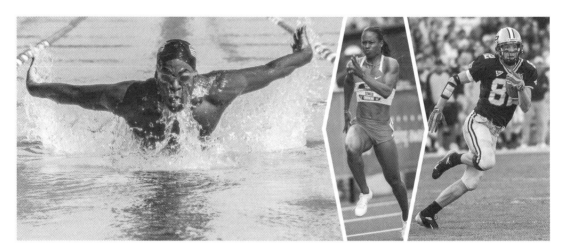

Different sports require different types of strength. Training in a particular strength zone produces strength and performance adaptations that are exclusive to the zone itself.

(a) ©StockByte; *(b)* and *(c)* © Human Kinetics

Table 4.1 STANDARD SPEEDS 1RM PERCENTAGE CORRELATION

VELOCITY (M/SEC)	RELATIONSHIP TO ESTIMATED 1RM
0.12-0.50	80%-100%
0.50-0.75	60%-80%
0.75-1.0	40%-60%
1.0-1.3	20%-40%
1.3+	Body weight-20%

While there are standard speeds that correlate to a 1RM percentage, as shown in table 4.1, it's really best to create your own ranges based on your clients. Figure 4.1 represents these ranges that work for my clients based on approximately 75 to 100 athletes who generally range from 16 to 25 years of age. Included is the correlation to a 1RM as well as the ranges for both upper- and lower-body movements. Because of a larger range of motion created by the longer limb lengths associated with the lower body (e.g., squats, deadlifts), speed ranges are an average of 0.10 to 0.15 meters per second lower on upper-body lifts (e.g., bench presses, rows).

Rigidity		Power		Elasticity

100% 90% 80%	70% 60%	50% 40%	30% 20%	10% 0%
Absolute strength	**Accelerative strength**	**Strength-speed (force)**	**Speed-strength (velocity)**	**Starting strength**
80%-100% 1RM	60%-80% 1RM	40%-60% 1RM	20%-40% 1RM	Bodyweight-20% 1RM

	Absolute strength	Accelerative strength	Strength-speed (force)	Speed-strength (velocity)	Starting strength
Lower-body speed ranges	<.50 m/s	.50-.75 m/s	.75-1.0 m/s	1.0-1.3 m/s	>1.3 m/s
Upper-body speed ranges	<.40 m/s	.40-.60 m/s	.60-.85 m/s	.85-1.1 m/s	>1.1 m/s

Figure 4.1 Special strength zones by speed.

Reprinted by permission from J.B. Mann, *Developing Explosive Athletes: Use of Velocity-Based Training in Athletes*, 3rd ed. (Muskegon, MI: Ultimate Athlete Concepts, 2016).

A CLOSER LOOK AT THE SPECIAL STRENGTH ZONES

The body only cares about the stimulus that is placed upon it. It is unaware of the type of exercise being done; it only knows "stress and stimulus." Let's take a look at these zones individually as well as what they mean in relation to the training adaptation that they help achieve and the best time in the training cycle to apply them.

Absolute Strength Zone

The absolute strength zone (0.10 to 0.50 meters per second), also known as maximal strength, is the range that athletes will see their 1RM fall into, but it will not necessarily be where an athlete performs best under heavy load due to the lack of a higher velocity component in the lift (see figure 4.2). Absolute strength, along with accelerative strength, is the primary strength adaptation when training with maximal strength (phase III, which is discussed in greater detail in chapter 9), and it is generally developed between one and four reps. While many coaches believe that you should train power capability all year round, they are missing the fact that power is a function of maximal strength, and to improve power initially, we must first improve maximal strength through training in the absolute strength zone.

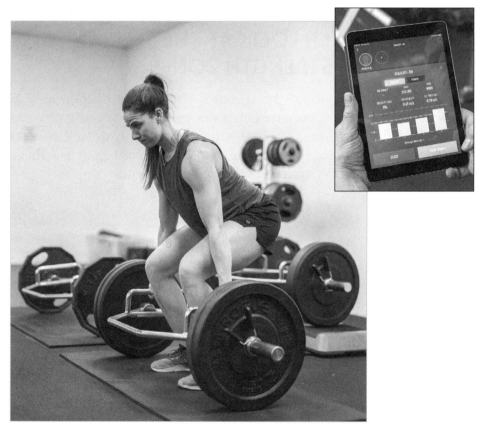

Figure 4.2 Training in the absolute strength zone with a deadlift at 80 to 100 percent 1RM.

The adaptation achieved is an increased diameter of the cross-sectional area of the high threshold muscle fibers and an increased number of motor units able to be recruited in a single effort (intramuscular coordination), thus improving the contractile properties of the muscle. Note, however, that more experienced lifters with larger cross-sectional areas of muscle fiber can use even lower "working" velocities and are able to better grind out reps (some as low as 0.10 meters per second) due to their higher levels of absolute strength. This is why performing a full force–velocity profile and establishing each athlete's true 1RM velocities will give us the most accurate ranges from person to person.

Although absolute strength is the foundation that all faster stimuli sit on, it is not the only capacity to develop. While all athletes, especially younger ones, need to start here, there is a point of diminishing returns when training for speed and elasticity becomes a priority.

EXERCISES

Compound exercises (exercises that use multiple joints at a time) such as squats, deadlifts, or bench press work best in this zone due to the ability to perform them under heavy loads while maintaining good form.

PROTOCOL

Number of exercises	2-3
Sets	4-8
Reps	1-4
Total reps	15-30 per body part
Intensity	> 80% 1RM
Rest	3-5 min, or as needed

TIME OF YEAR

Early to middle off-season

Accelerative Strength Zone

The accelerative strength zone (0.50 to 0.75 meters per second) is known as accelerative strength (or submaximal strength, as it is referred to in the following chapters) and is described as moving a moderately heavy load at a moderate speed (see figure 4.3). This zone is typically where an athlete's best force output is done, especially when load is between approximately 0.65 to 0.75 meters per second or 60 to 65 percent 1RM. This is due to the fact that we are still using heavy enough loads to create a strength adaptation, but they are light enough to allow athletes to move their body and the bar quick enough to enhance the acceleration side of the force equation (force = mass × acceleration). This accelerative strength zone is a workhorse because it serves many different training adaptations and is used with absolute strength—not only in phase III (see chapter 9) but also in phase IV (see chapter 10)—to train alactic power and to maintain both strength and power

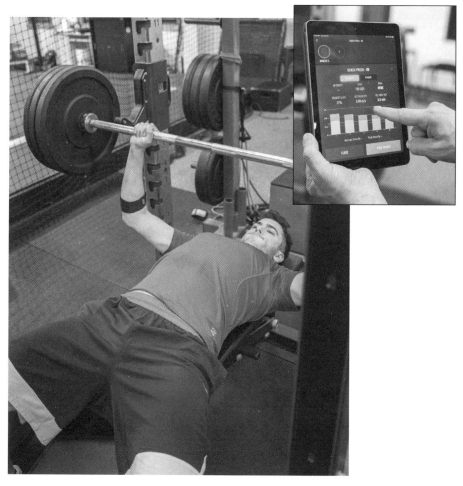

Figure 4.3 Training in the accelerative strength zone with a bench press at 60 to 80 percent 1RM.

throughout the competitive period (in-season) as the season progresses. (This and the training phases are covered in detail in part III.)

The ability to move the bar or body more quickly enables athletes to create more peak force than at heavier loads because of the quicker time component used. During the in-season, this becomes the trait that diminishes the most quickly (7 to 10 days) and must be maintained. This zone is where I generally like to start athletes because we focus on intermuscular coordination, which basically is the coordination within different muscles and groups of muscles to perform a specific movement. This helps with priming the nervous system and mastering the movement due to less stress on the system and joints from using lighter loads. Intermuscular coordination goes a long way in being more successful when higher loads (maximal strength) are introduced.

EXERCISES

Exercises that are used in the absolute strength zone can also be used in the accelerative strength zone, but they are performed at a lower percentage of the athlete's 1RM. This is done in order to add a higher acceleration component to the training.

PROTOCOL

Number of exercises	2-3
Sets	4-10
Reps	3-8
Total reps	16-40 per body part
Intensity	60%-80% 1RM
Rest	1-3 min, or as needed

TIME OF YEAR

Early and late off-season and in-season (maintenance)

Strength-Speed and Speed-Strength Zones

For years, these two zones, where power lives, have been somewhat of a gray area because sport scientists and researchers were unable to discern the split between strength-speed and speed-strength based on a percentage of a 1RM (Mann 2016). For this reason, when training in the strength-speed and speed-strength zones, using a load that displays the greatest amount of power as expressed in watts on the device rather than velocity seems to work best for me. Athletes with thicker cross-sectional areas of muscle fiber (rigidity) possess a higher potential for force output, but there is a cost associated with this. Thicker tissues are less elastic, making it harder to stretch the muscle, much like a really thick rubber band. This generally coincides with strength-speed or strength-power velocities. Athletes with greater contractile properties (elasticity) are generally better at moving faster and are more comfortable training on the velocity side of power, which is speed-strength or speed-power (see figure 4.4). However, their smaller muscle cross-sectional area limits muscular force production capabilities compared to the thicker, more rigid athlete, making them less equipped to stand up against heavy loads. See figure 4.4 for traits of these two types of athlete.

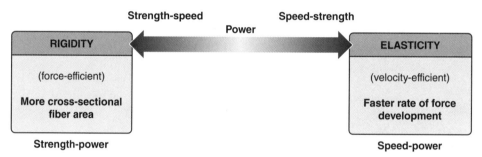

Figure 4.4 Differences in traits between athletes with rigid or elastic tissue properties.

In addition, when training for power, it is also important to take into consideration velocity loss. When velocity loss becomes greater than 10 to 15 percent from set to set, the athlete is no longer training power and, therefore, the load needs to be decreased (see chapter 6). Now, with VBT, we are able to monitor not only velocity to better separate the two but also power output, as well as prescribe the appropriate method based on where an athlete can perform better—the force side of power (strength-power) or the velocity side of power (speed-power). (The force–velocity profile is covered further in chapter 9.)

Strength-Speed Zone

Force is what moves us, so if you don't have adequate force production, you're not going to create optimal power. Strength-speed is described as moving a moderately heavy load as fast as possible. The strength-speed zone (0.75 to 1.0 meters per second) sits on and trains the "force side" of power on the curve. It is the zone where a more force-efficient athlete likes to live when it comes to producing the highest rate of force development (see figure 4.5). This zone's protocol (load) requires near-maximum to moderate muscular contractions, with a secondary emphasis on the rate of production (velocity).

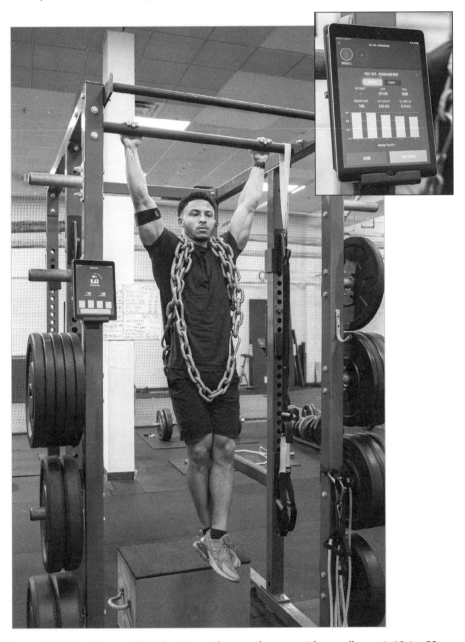

Figure 4.5 Training within the strength-speed zone with a pull-up at 40 to 60 percent 1RM.

It is important to note, however, that strength-speed often requires the use of bands for accommodating resistance and assistance. Band *resistance* reduces much of the deceleration component associated with lifting lighter loads, allowing velocity-efficient athletes to accelerate for a longer period of time and achieve higher force outputs. Band *assistance* improves the contractile properties of the muscles in force-efficient athletes. (Review acceleration and deceleration in chapter 2.)

EXERCISES

Weighted jumps, band-assisted or band-resisted bench press, deadlifts, squats

PROTOCOL

Number of exercises	1-2
Sets	4-10
Reps	3-5 (use the maximum amount of reps that allow power output, which is based on velocity or power loss, to remain under 10%-15% from set to set)
Total reps	18-36 per body part
Intensity	40%-60% 1RM, or wherever peak power lies in watts
Rest	Depends on work–rest ratios conducive to individual sport

TIME OF YEAR

Late off-season or preseason

Speed-Strength Zone

While some athletes sit on the strength side of power, others live more on the velocity side of power. Speed-strength, or speed-power, as it is referred to in the following chapters, is described as moving a lighter weight as fast as possible. The speed-strength zone's (1.0 to 1.3 meters per second) protocol is where rate of force production, or velocity, takes precedence over force, making load secondary in nature (see figure 4.6). This zone has a prime emphasis on speed, and it is where a more velocity-efficient athlete likes to live when it comes to producing the highest rate of power.

It is also important to note that speed-strength often requires the use of either accommodating resistance or assistance such as bands. Band resistance can be used in order to take out much of the deceleration component that is associated with lifting lighter loads. This will allow athletes that are more "velocity efficient" to

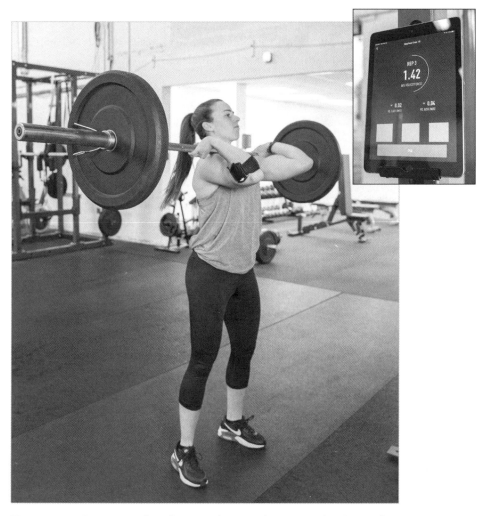

Figure 4.6 Training within the speed-strength zone with a hang clean at 20 to 40 percent 1RM.

accelerate for a longer period of time and help achieve higher force outputs while band assistance can be used to assist and improve the contractile properties of the muscles in athletes that are more "force- efficient" (please review acceleration and deceleration in chapter 2).

EXERCISES

Olympic lifts, weighted jumps with lighter loads than used for strength-speed, medicine ball throws, and various forms of plyometrics

PROTOCOL

Number of exercises	1-2
Sets	4-10
Reps	3-5 (use the maximum amount of reps that allows power output, based on velocity or power loss, to remain >10% from set to set)
Total reps	25-45 per body part
Intensity	20%-40%, or wherever peak power lies in watts
Rest	Depends on work–rest ratios conducive to individual sport

As mentioned previously, at this velocity, I like to incorporate Olympic lifts, such as hang cleans and snatches, which are ballistic in nature due the fact that force is imparted on the bar for only a short moment (until the second pull) before the implement is projected into the air. As a result, these types of exercises are generally calculated using peak concentric velocity (see chapter 2) and do not fall in these general ranges provided. Using mean velocities to calculate ballistic movements will give us inaccurate readings: There is no deceleration phase because the lifter is not trying to lock or grind out a rep.

When it comes to Olympic lifts, another variable needs to be considered: height. The taller the athlete, the longer the lever arm—and the greater the abilities to both develop force over a longer period of time (i.e., "distance") and produce higher velocities. This is not unlike the difference in speeds between upper- and lower-body lifts that was discussed earlier in this chapter. This metric is important to consider when training multiple athletes in a group setting. If taller athletes are trying to pull the same slower tempos as their shorter counterparts over a further distance, *overtraining* is more likely to be the main adaptation achieved.

The following table provides velocity ranges for two Olympic lifts (snatches and hang cleans) based on athlete heights that I have been using over the past few years. I have converted heights from meters to feet and inches.

Olympic lift	Athlete height	Velocity (m/sec)
Snatch	5'0"-5'2"	1.6
	5'3"-5'6"	1.85
	5'7"-5'10"	2.1
	5'11"-6'1"	2.3
	6'2"-6'4"	2.5
	>6'4"	2.7
Hang clean	5'0"-5'2"	1.55
	5'3"-5'6"	1.62
	5'7"-6'0"	1.7
	6'1"-6'4"	1.85
	>6'4"	2.0

Calculations are based on information supplied by Dr. Bryan Mann.

TIME OF YEAR

Late off-season or preseason

Starting Strength (Speed) Zone

The starting strength (speed) zone (greater than 1.3 meters per second) is best described as the ability to overcome inertia from a dead stop, such as a pitcher starting down the mound out of his glute load or a running back coming out of the "set" position and generally involves some sort of throwing, sprinting, or fast SSC plyometrics (see figure 4.7). Note that there is a misconception among many strength and conditioning coaches that the big core lifts, such as deadlifts, will help improve starting strength. These core lifts are more designed to train absolute strength.

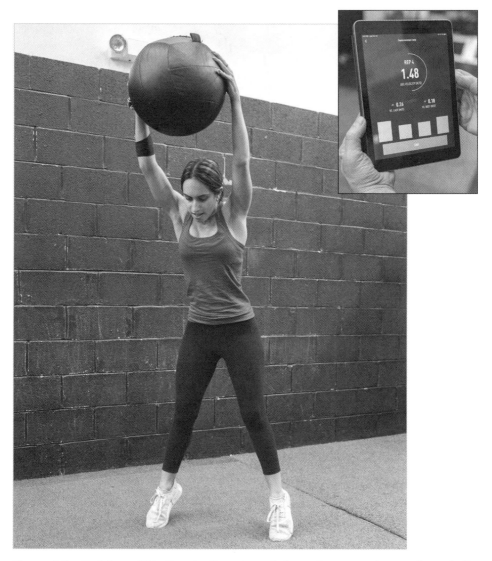

Figure 4.7 Training within the starting strength (speed) zone with a medicine ball slam at body weight to 20 percent 1RM.

EXERCISES

Medicine ball throws; exercises that use weighted implements, such as weighted vests, balls, javelin, discus (track and field), and ropes

PROTOCOL

Number of exercises	2-3
Sets	4-8
Reps	5-12 (use the maximum amount of reps that allows power output, based on velocity loss, to remain >5%-10% from set to set)
Total reps	40-84 per body part
Intensity	Between body weight (no extra load) and 20%, or wherever peak power lies in watts
Rest	Enough to ensure power output stays within 10% from set to set

TIME OF YEAR

Preseason

Figure 4.8 sums up the different types of strength used in training athletes as well as which part of the curve they used while training. Accelerative strength is not included, but it would fall between maximal (absolute) strength and strength-speed. It is important to understand where on the force–velocity curve they are applied in order to be sure we are prescribing the correct type of strength for the adaptation we are looking for.

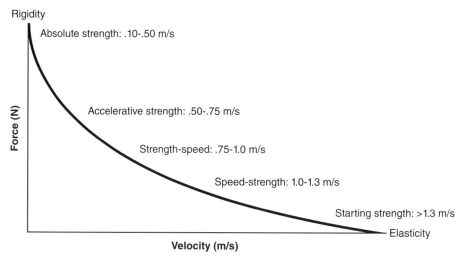

Rigidity

Absolute strength: .10-.50 m/s

Accelerative strength: .50-.75 m/s

Strength-speed: .75-1.0 m/s

Speed-strength: 1.0-1.3 m/s

Starting strength: >1.3 m/s

Elasticity

Force (N)

Velocity (m/s)

Figure 4.8 The types of strength and where they fall on the force–velocity curve.

Different athletes require different types of strength based on the sport they play as well as the time of the year. When using VBT, we are able to better pinpoint those strengths, whether they are absolute strength, accelerative strength, or speed-strength (power), with greater accuracy than by simply using a percentage of a standard 1RM. This allows both the coach and athlete to use the S.A.I.D. principle and target the specific adaptation that they are training in that specific training block.

CHAPTER 5

Calculating a One-Rep Max

This chapter provides a discussion on some methods for calculating 1RM using VBT and includes an explanation for what force–velocity profiling, also known as load profiling, is and how it relates to training. We look at the step-by-step process for creating a force–velocity profile prior to the calculation of an athlete's true 1RM. In addition, we discuss mean velocity threshold, or rep-to-failure (RTF) testing.

THE IMPORTANCE OF ONE-REP MAXIMUM TESTING

A 1RM is the maximum amount of weight that a person can possibly lift for one repetition (see figure 5.1). For years, the 1RM has been the industry standard used for determining maximal strength and the upper limit when seeking the desired load for an exercise, (i.e., a percentage of the 1RM when seeking a specific training adaptation). The 1RM is both a desirable tool when programming and a great marker for improvements in strength in any serious athlete's lifting protocol.

Every exercise has a different 1RM, so testing must be done on each exercise within the athlete's training program. For example, a breakdown of workloads for absolute strength and accelerative strength that are based on percentages of this 1RM for an athlete with a recorded

300-pound (136 kg) 1RM in the back squat and a 220-pound (100 kg) 1RM in the bench press would look something like this:

Back Squat

Working weight and absolute strength: 300 pounds (load) × 0.85 (percentage) = 255 pounds (136 kg × 0.85 = 116 kg)

Working weight and accelerative strength: 300 pounds (load) × 0.60 (percentage) = 180 pounds (136 kg × 0.60 = 82 kg)

Bench Press

Working weight and absolute strength: 220 pounds (load) × 0.90 (percentage) = 198 pounds (100 kg × 0.90 = 90 kg)

Working weight and accelerative strength: 220 pounds (load) × 0.75 (percentage) = 165 pounds (100 kg × 0.75 = 75 kg)

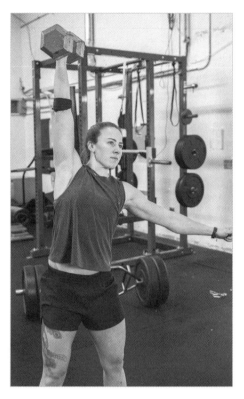

Figure 5.1 Accelerometers (or LPTs) can be used to calculate a 1RM using VBT. Just be sure to be consistent with the device when testing and again when retesting.

THE LOAD–VELOCITY RELATIONSHIP

A recent study found a strong correlation between velocity and corresponding percentages of a 1RM (Jidovtseff, et al. 2009). Another study found the average percentage to be a 0.00-0.01 meters per second variation between mean velocity and a true 1RM, which demonstrates the near-perfect correlation between percentages of a 1RM and the corresponding velocity (González-Badillo and Sánchez-Medina 2010). In my opinion, this recent information has broken a lot of ground in terms of the reliability

When calculating a 1RM with VBT, as the load increases, the movement velocity decreases.

of using VBT when calculating a 1RM. If you recall, in chapter 4, table 4.1 shows how velocity speed can correlate to a 1RM. That same table (table 5.1) can also demonstrate how VBT works into the load–velocity relationship. When calculating a 1RM with VBT, as the load increases, the movement velocity decreases.

Table 5.1 VELOCITY–1RM CORRELATION

VELOCITY (M/SEC)	RELATIONSHIP TO ESTIMATED 1RM
0.12-0.25	95%-100%
0.25-0.50	80%-95%
0.50-0.75	60%-80%
0.75-1.0	40%-60%
1.0-1.3	20%-40%

Table 5.2 provides the approximate corresponding velocity to a load's percentage when using VBT for the same 300-pound (136 kg). It is an approximation because, remember, VBT numbers vary slightly from athlete to athlete. This simply includes a range based on special strength zones previously discussed (see figure 4.1 in chapter 4).

Table 5.2 EXAMPLE OF LOAD–VELOCITY RELATIONSHIP FOR A 300-POUND (136 KG) 1RM

LOAD	PERCENTAGE (1RM)	WORKING WEIGHT	VBT VELOCITY (M/SEC)
300 lb (136 kg)	300 × 0.85 (136 × 0.85)	255 lb (116 kg)	0.40-.050
300 lb (136 kg)	300 × 0.60 (136 × 0.60)	180 lb (82 kg)	0.65-0.75

1RM TESTING METHODS

As you recall from chapter 3, both LPTs and accelerometers can be used to calculate a 1RM. I use both on a daily basis just to ensure consistency with each device for multiple testings and retesting. Accelerometers' algorithms can make measurements slightly skewed, and some accelerometers are more dependable than others. Just make sure that your method of measuring stays the same throughout the entire testing process.

There are many different methods for testing and calculating a 1RM using VBT. However, for the purpose of this book, I include only the two

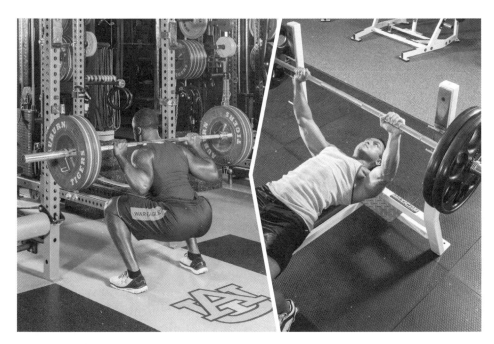

Every exercise has a different 1RM, so testing must be done on each exercise within the athlete's training program.

(a) and *(b)* © Human Kinetics

methods I use to calculate 1RMs: velocity profile and RTF test. Regardless the method you use, keep in mind the following:

- *Velocity is inconsistent and less stable at lighter loads.* The heavier the load is, the more accurate the 1RM prediction becomes. Velocity is less stable at lighter loads (less than 60 percent 1RM) because the faster the movement becomes, the need to decelerate that movement increases. Therefore, mean propulsive velocity is a better metric to use in this circumstance because it measures only the accelerative phase.

- *Each device measures velocity in different ways.* Different devices may produce slightly distinct calculations. This is okay, but again, it is important to be sure that the unit is consistent and the measuring protocol is kept the same when retesting.

Velocity Profile

Recording velocities at different percentages of an athlete's 1RM makes the numbers more customized to that specific athlete. A velocity profile contains the recorded velocities of loads that are moved at various percentages of a 1RM. The beauty of a velocity profile is that once you have the velocities of a certain percentage of your 1RM, they can be used instead of the percentage itself. For example, if I move 75 percent of my 1RM at 0.60 meters per second, I can now use 0.60 meters per second as my loading intensity rather than 75 percent. More importantly, as we discussed earlier, 1RMs can fluctuate by as much as 18 percent day to day, so using velocity will take these fluctuations into consideration and prevent over- or undertraining for a given day. And it goes without saying that it is also important to monitor trends in your athletes.

A velocity profile contains the recorded velocities of loads that are moved at various percentages of a 1RM.

It is important to note that, while strength may vary among athletes, the corresponding velocities do not (Mann 2016). In other words, we can have two athletes who vary greatly in strength and have two completely different 1RMs in the squat. However, when working at 60 percent of each athlete's 1RM, both will pull at the relatively same velocity (see table 5.3).

Table 5.3 COMPARISON OF TWO ATHLETES WITH DIFFERENT 1RMS FOR THE SQUAT

	LOAD	PERCENTAGE (60% 1RM)	WORKING WEIGHT	VBT VELOCITY (M/SEC)
Athlete 1	300 lb (126 kg)	300 × 0.60 (126)	180 lb (76 kg)	0.79
Athlete 2	475 lb (215 kg)	475 × 0.60 (215)	285 lb (129 kg)	0.76

Performing a Velocity Profile

The following section describes the step-by-step procedure I use when creating a force (load)–velocity profile for my athletes. In this particular example, I use a back squat; however, this same protocol can be applied for every exercise using VBT for an athlete's program. It takes the athlete through the various loads on the way to a 1RM. The loads can then be calculated when training at specific percentages throughout the year in order to effectively target those specific strength zones. You can use the given ranges from table 5.1, but a velocity profile is much more precise to the exact load for the particular athlete you are working with.

Before performing the profile, athletes must be weighed wearing light-weight shorts and a top (or sports bra), with shoes and any accessories removed. Taking weigh measurements is important for establishing a baseline weight that is entered into the unit or the app in order to get accurate power outputs for the lifts. A baseline weight is also a good way to show progress in lean body mass throughout the training process. With the LPT, zero out the unit according to instructions to allow for

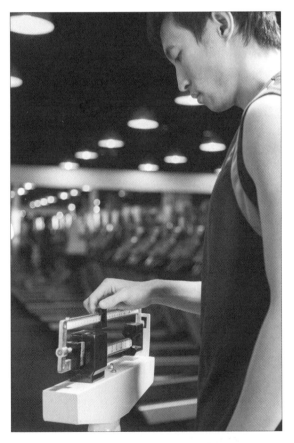

Weighing the athlete is important for establishing a baseline weight that is then entered into the unit or the app. This ensures that accurate power outputs on the lifts are given and progress in lean body mass is shown throughout the training process.

FangXiaNuo/E+/Getty Images

adjustments to angles. If using an accelerometer, place the band on either the forearm or the bar, whichever one the manufacturer recommends.

I use a 16-inch (41 cm) box to keep the depth of the back squat the same from rep to rep. While this does take away a bit of eccentric load and elasticity, I feel that most sports never use a stretch deeper than 16 inches (41 cm). It is okay to use a lower box, however, if that feels appropriate. Whatever you use to test, make sure it is constant from athlete to athlete and when reassessing.

Performing a short general warm-up promotes blood flow and increases body temperature. Next, a more specific warm-up prepares the body for the exercise being tested. In this example, we are testing the back squat, so the specific warm-up starts with performing back squats for sets of triples (3 reps) until a velocity of 1.0-1.2 meters per second (approximately 45 to 50 percent 1RM) is achieved. Then, the profile begins, as follows:

Rest

90 seconds between sets

Reps

- Triples (3 reps) until 0.75 meters per second (approximately 60 percent 1RM) is achieved
- Doubles (2 reps) until 0.50 meters per second (approximately 80 percent 1RM) is achieved
- Singles (1 rep) to failure (100 percent 1RM)

We generally look for increments from 0.05 to no more than 0.07 meters per second from set to set. Moving up in 10- to 20-pound increments (5 to 9 kg) is a good approach when loads start to reach 0.50 (80 percent) 1RM; however, at the beginning of the profile, when loads are lighter, you may need these increments to be higher (sometimes even as much as 30 to 40 pounds [14 to 18 kg] and even higher prior to 1.0 meter per second). It all depends on the athlete's ability.

Only the concentric portion of the lift is measured, so using a comfortable, controlled eccentric (lowering) of the bar or body is important to ensure that the athlete is not lowering the load too quickly for obvious safety reasons. This is especially true as the loads increase to higher levels or are moved too slowly, negatively affecting activation in the concentric portion of the lift. See figure 5.2 for an example of the back squat being performed.

Note that, at lighter weights, there may be some extra movement at the squat lockout with the load still being so light (see figure 5.3). This will not affect data if using peak velocity (PV) because that portion of

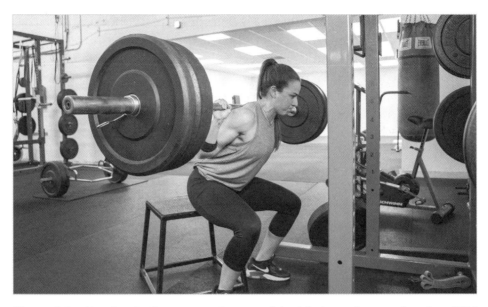

Figure 5.2 Keeping testing parameters consistent is key when performing 1RM testing. Here, a 16-inch (41 cm) box is used to control depth from rep to rep.

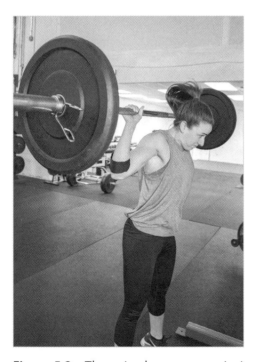

Figure 5.3 The extra bar movement at lockout compromises accuracy when using mean velocities.

the movement has already been calculated. It will, however, have some effect on the mean velocity because it allows the bar a longer period of time to produce more force and velocity. This will not be the case as the weight gets heavier (above 60 percent).

Sample Force–Velocity Profile

Table 5.4 features a 40-minute load–velocity profile I performed on a 5 foot 11 inch, 180-pound (180 cm, 82 kg) male ice hockey player with an estimated 1RM of 375 pounds (170 kg) for the back squat. Because of his higher training age (roughly four to five years of lifting experience), we were able to perform a full profile with many data points, taking him all the way down to his true 1RM. We now have a full velocity profile for this athlete with speeds that are specific to him alone. As I previously mentioned, this is more accurate than using ranges, but it is not always possible when working with groups.

Obviously, the closer we can get to a 1RM (usually somewhere between 0.17 meters per second and 0.30 meters per second) makes our results more accurate. However, with novice athletes who have a much younger training age, I typically take them to only 0.50 to .60 meters per second (roughly 75 to 80 percent 1RM) and approximate an estimated 1RM from there. This has a much better risk–reward than to cause inexperienced athletes to fail in the weight room both physically and psychologically. An example for an estimated 300-pound (136 kg) 1RM would look like this:

240 lb (109 kg) back squat @ 0.50 (80%) = 300 lb est. 1RM

(300 lb [136 kg] × 0.80 = 240 lb [109 kg])

Table 5.4 SAMPLE VELOCITY PROFILE FOR AN ICE HOCKEY PLAYER WITH AN ESTIMATED 1RM OF 375 POUNDS (170 KG)

	LOAD	VBT VELOCITY (M/SEC)
Warm-up	95 lb (43 kg)	1.32
	110 lb (50 kg)	1.26
	150 lb (68 kg)	1.15
Triples: strength–speed (40%-60% 1RM)	170 lb (77 kg)	1.03
	175 lb (79 kg)	0.97
	185 lb (84 kg)	0.87
	195 lb (88 kg)	0.81
	205 lb (93 kg)	0.78
Doubles: accelerative strength (60%-80% 1RM)	225 lb (102 kg)	0.75
	245 lb (111 kg)	0.70
	265 lb (120 kg)	0.64
	280 lb (127 kg)	0.59
	300 lb (136 kg)	0.54
Singles: maximal strength (80%-100% 1RM)	315 lb (143 kg)	0.48
	330 lb (150 kg)	0.42
	345 lb (156 kg)	0.32
	355 lb (161 kg)	0.27
	365 lb (166 kg)	0.24
	375 lb (170 kg)	0.21 (last rep 100% 1RM)

Repetition-to-Failure Test

If time constraints (such as with groups) are an issue, or if I want to acquire a 1RM velocity without a profile, I will take the athlete through the method known as the repetition-to-failure (RTF) test, which takes the athlete to their minimal velocity threshold (MVT). An MVT is the mean concentric velocity (MCV) produced during the last successful repetition of a set and another way to acquire velocity for a 1RM. This could be during the 1RM itself, or alternatively, the velocity produced from the last successful repetition during an RTF test.

RTF testing starts as if you are performing a load–velocity profile, except you stop when the athlete meets a measured velocity of around 0.65 meters per second or approximately 70 percent 1RM. Then, you have the athlete take the next set to failure (as many reps as possible). Note that for the RTF test, I like to use 70 percent 1RM instead of the 60 percent 1RM usually used by other practitioners because I can still put less stress on the joints from lighter load than a traditional 1RM, but I do not have to perform as many reps as I would at 60 percent 1RM. This helps avoid failure caused by fatigue. One study has shown that both a failure on true 1RM and an MVT resulting from an RTF test will result in nearly the same velocity (Izquierdo et al. 2006). Using the same ice hockey player from the earlier full velocity profile, table 5.5 compares the athlete's true 1RM velocity and his estimated 1RM by using RTF.

Table 5.5 COMPARING VELOCITY READINGS FROM A TRUE 1RM AND A RTF TEST WITH AN ESTIMATED 1RM OF 375 POUNDS (170 KG)

METHOD	LOAD PER REP	1RM VELOCITY (M/SEC)
Velocity profile (true 1RM)	375 lb (175 kg) × 1	0.021
RTF (minimal velocity threshold)	265 lb (120 kg) (to failure)	0.023

Training athletes year-round can be like trying to hit a moving target. The various situations that occur between in-season and off-season both on and off the field require training different traits at different times specific to each athlete. It is why velocity profiling is such an extremely valuable tool for any athlete or coach. Providing athletes individualized data through profiling and using VBT helps with pinpointing these adaptations more quickly while taking day-to-day fluctuations into consideration and giving athletes the best chance for success in their respective sport. And remember: Always make sure that your LPT or accelerometer is giving you consistent, dependable information every time.

Using Autoregulation and Velocity Loss

This chapter presents the concepts and principles of using autoregulation and discusses how using VBT can maximize each session through monitoring recovery and fatigue to help avoid under- or overtraining. We also look at various methods that use velocity loss to achieve different training adaptations when training power as well as some quick tests that test the central nervous system's (CNS) readiness daily.

DEFINING FATIGUE AND AUTOREGULATION

Fatigue experienced during exercise can be defined as the "inability to maintain a given exercise intensity and can vary with the nature of the activity (intensity and duration), the athlete's training status, and the present environmental conditions" (Brooks et al 2004).

The brain and spinal cord make up CNS (see figure 6.1). The somatic nervous system transmits sensory and motor signals to and from the CNS. The efficient routing of these motor signals must be in place to achieve optimal performance and efficient technique. Famed performance coach Charlie Francis (1982) defines the CNS as "the optimal transmitter of nervous signals and motor pathways."

Francis describes CNS fatigue as the "by-products of high-intensity exercise[s that] build up to a point where the CNS impulses (necessary to contract the muscle fibers) are handicapped." Most studies involving CNS fatigue have been done using endurance exercise rather than examining CNS function when training speed and power in a high-performance

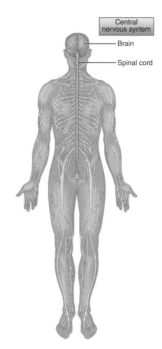

Figure 6.1 The central nervous system: the optimal transmitter from the brain to the muscles and skeletal system.

athlete. According to Francis, the following primarily causes this drop in function in explosive athletes:

- High-intensity work occurring too frequently in a training cycle
- Too much high-intensity volume in a single training session
- Introducing high-intensity training too rapidly into a training program when residual fatigue still exists

When we train, we must consider changes in readiness caused by this stress or fatigue, and not just the stress from training alone, but all stressors. Hans Selye stated in his book *The Stress of Life* (1956) that "all stressors draw from the same pool." So, whether it is game play, weight training, school, relationships or a rough night out on the town, stress needs to be monitored and training adjusted accordingly. This is otherwise known as autoregulation, and it is one of the great advantages to using VBT.

Traditionally, resistance-training intensity has been derived from a percentage of an athlete's 1RM. More recently, however, a study has shown that practically perfect correlations ($r = 0.95$) were observed in the relationship between load–velocity and a predicted 1RM (Jidovtseff

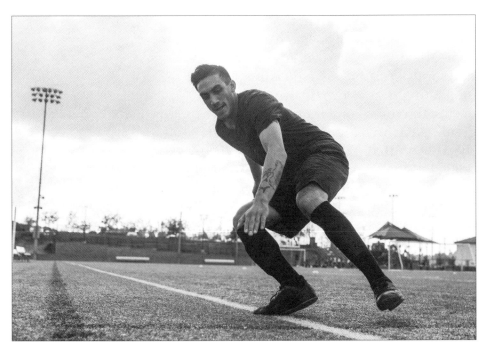

Introducing high-intensity work such as shuttle runs too frequently or too early in an athlete's training program can reduce CNS output considerably.

The Good Brigade/DigitalVision/Getty Images

et al. 2011). This makes VBT an extremely reliable and more convenient alternative than the traditional percentage-based 1RM. It enables both the coach and the athlete to match established resisting training variables, such as the percentage of an athlete's 1RM, to specific movement velocities. Doing so helps them objectively identify the onset of neuromuscular fatigue so they can gauge training readiness.

Another study found that, based on these daily stressors, an athlete's 1RMs can change by as much as +/- 18 percent from day to day (Flanagan and Jovanovic 2014). While I have used the traditional percentage-based 1RM protocol for years and still do sometimes, I have seen firsthand the ease of use as well as the ability to take day-to-day fatigue into account by monitoring velocity instead of load. The decline in velocity across a number of sets or reps can tell us the amount of muscle stress or teardown. This is especially useful when monitoring fatigue for several athletes in a group setting (see figure 6.2).

When we train, we must consider changes in readiness caused by this stress or fatigue, and not just the stress from training alone, but all stressors.

The use of autoregulation allows athletes to train using loads that are appropriate for their specific readiness for *that particular day*, meaning, despite highs and lows in strength during the course of a training program, the correlated percentage of the 1RM to that particular velocity does not change (Sánchez-Medina and González-Badillo 2011). In other words, if you move 70 percent 1RM at 0.62 meters per second, this velocity will always relate to 70 percent 1RM even if strength gains go up or down.

To further explain this point, table 6.1 provides details of three separate workouts for an athlete who has been profiled with a 285-pound (129 kg) 1RM for the split squat during the athlete's initial testing. For the first workout, the athlete moves 200 pounds (91 kg) at 0.62 meters per second, which is approximately 70

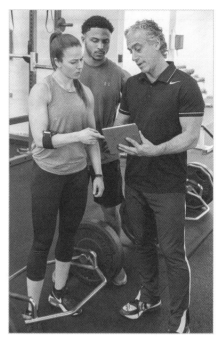

Figure 6.2 Using VBT to monitor velocity loss instead of load is especially helpful when working with groups.

percent 1RM (285 pounds [129 kg] × 0.70 = 200 pounds [91 kg]). During the next workout, the athletes seems to be affected by outside stressors such as a lack of sleep or hydration and moves only 175 pounds (79 kg) at 0.62 meters per second, which is still 70 percent 1RM *for this particular day*. This now equates to a 250 pounds (113 kg) 1RM (250 pounds [113 kg] × 0.70 = 175 pounds [79 kg]) and signifies a 12-percent *decrease* in this athlete's 1RM from residual stress and accumulated fatigue. Simply plowing through day 1's numbers could increase the likelihood of injury. Then, on the other hand, after sleeping well that night and then acing finals the next day, this athlete comes in feeling exuberant and pulls 210 pounds (95 kg) at 0.62 meters per second for a third workout. Because we base intensity on speed, we know that this is still 70 percent 1RM that now equates to a 300-pound (136 kg) 1RM (300 pounds [136 kg] × 0.70 = 210 pounds [95 kg]). This indicates a five-percent *increase* in this athlete's 1RM—the kind of day we all hope for!

If we just based every training session on this athlete's initial 1RM test, we would be not only overtraining this athlete on day 2 when training

Table 6.1 DAILY TRAINING READINESS FLUCTUATIONS FOR AN ATHLETE WITH AN ESTIMATED 285-POUND (129 KG) 1RM

TRAINING DAY	LOAD (3 REPS)	AVERAGE VELOCITY (M/SEC PER SET)	DAILY ESTIMATED 1RM
Day 1	200 lb (91 kg)	0.62	285 lb (129 kg)
Day 2	175 lb (79 kg)	0.61	250 lb (113 kg)
Day 3	210 lb (95 kg)	0.63	300 lb (136 kg)

readiness was lower but also increasing the athlete's risk for possible injury. Sánchez-Medina and González-Badillo (2011) found that a high correlation between velocity loss and the metabolic stress (lactate and ammonia accumulation) stems from overtraining (fatigue). And, on day 3 when training readiness was high, we would be both undertraining the athlete and likely impeding training adaptation and progress. This is a terrific example of VBT's extraordinary power for autoregulating training and maximizing gains for your athletes.

TARGETING STRENGTH ADAPTATIONS THROUGH VELOCITY-LOSS MONITORING

When training with VBT, percentage of velocity loss can be monitored using an LPT or accelerometer. Each device can be set to signify losses in power output (measured in watts) between reps or from set to set (the more popular method) when training for power and power endurance (see figure 6.3). When work reaches the prescribed velocity or power loss, the athlete has the option to lower the weight, increase rest time, or end the workout altogether.

Pareja-Blanco and colleagues (2016) found that the progressive buildup of muscle fatigue caused by a more pronounced repetition velocity loss is an important variable to exercise stimulus for resistance training concerning its influence on functional and structural neuromuscular changes in strength, power, and hypertrophy. Monitoring these losses is crucial to chasing specific training adaptations as well as ensuring we are not creating any residual soreness that may negatively affect upcoming games or event performances. Table 6.2 shows three different training adaptations based on repetition velocity losses within a set according to this study. (We will take a closer look at these parameters in the later chapters on programming.)

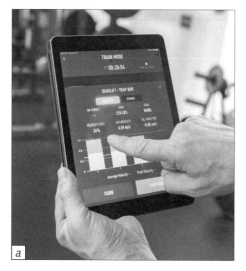 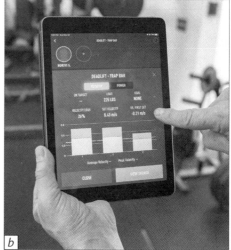

Figure 6.3 Losses in velocity can be monitored (a) between reps or (b) from set to set when training for endurance.

Table 6.2 VELOCITY LOSS AS ASSOCIATED WITH SPECIFIC TRAINING ADAPTATIONS

TRAINING ADAPTATION	VELOCITY LOSS
Hypertrophy I	40%-50%
Hypertrophy II	10%-20%
Strength	20%-30%
Power or speed	<10%

Hypertrophy I and II

When training hypertrophy I, higher drop-offs of 40 to 50 percent from rep to rep or from set to set elicit greater increases in the cross-sectional area of the type I (slow-twitch) muscle fibers, while drop-offs of 10 to 20 percent should be used for hypertrophy of the type II (fast-twitch) muscle fibers (hypertrophy II). To achieve hypertrophy I, athletes should use around 50 to 70 percent 1RM (or slightly less), which raises rep sets and increases time under tension, eliciting greater muscle damage. This, in turn, helps stimulate super compensation, resulting in the adaptive rebound above baseline after fatigue and recovery (rest). It allows the athlete to handle the same training load or an even greater load in

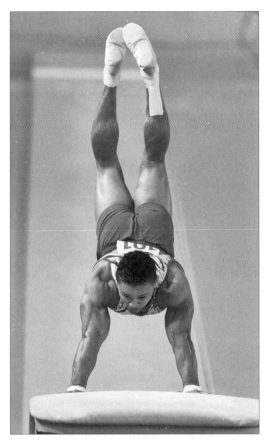

Monitoring losses is crucial to chasing specific training adaptations as well as ensuring we are not creating any residual soreness that may negatively affect next-day game or event performance.

LUIS ROBAYO/AFP via Getty Images

subsequent workouts if recovery is adequate and the new stress is timed properly. This stimulus is key to creating greater training adaptations that increases the cross-sectional area of just the type I muscle fibers.

However, if the goal is hypertrophy II of the fast-twitch (type II) muscle fibers (more on this in chapter 8), it is better to stay with a 10- to 20-percent drop-off in order to still elicit some teardown of the type I fibers while still maintaining stimulation of

When training hypertrophy I and II, higher drop-offs of 40 to 50 percent and 10 to 20 percent respectively from rep to rep or from set to set elicit the greatest increases in the cross-sectional area of the type I and type II muscle fibers.

the type II fibers (by keeping velocity losses lower than the 30 percent required to develop the type I fibers as described for hypertrophy I). This is important to remember because velocity losses greater than 40 percent or training to failure can severely limit jumping capabilities, resulting in direct onset muscle soreness (DOMS) for as much as 48 hours later. Note, however, that research has shown that the traditional approach of training to repetition failure does not necessarily lead to greater increases in strength or hypertrophy because an athlete's strength and readiness changes daily based on various stressors both in the weight room and outside of it (Pareja-Blanco et. al. 2020).

Strength

Contrary to popular belief, strength gains are significantly higher when lower velocity losses are used. As mentioned previously, a recent study showed that, while there were significant gains in hypertrophy, there were significant decreases in early rate of force development when athletes trained with velocity-loss thresholds above 30 percent (Pareja-Blanco et al. 2020). With this in mind, I like to use more submaximal loads (60 to 70 percent 1RM, or 0.60 to 0.75 meters per second) for multiple sets of three to five reps. Using a submaximal load to train strength with a high-set to low-rep–scheme ensures a moderate amount of velocity loss (20 to 30 percent), consistent rates of force development from set to set, and recovery within 24 to 48 hours. This is key to preventing residual soreness that may affect next-day performance.

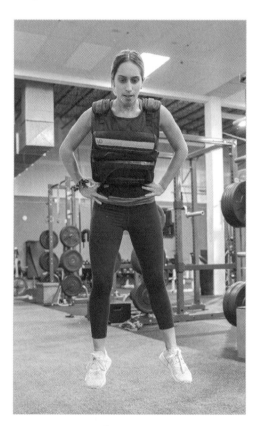

Figure 6.4 When training power and speed, it's imperative that athletes are not in a fatigued state because fatigue makes them unable to efficiently summon the needed type II muscle fibers required to be truly explosive.

Power and Speed

When training power and speed, it's imperative that athletes are not fatigued, otherwise they will be unable to efficiently summon the type II muscle fibers required to be explosive in the exercises (see figure 6.4). Training in a fatigued state can also create bad habits due to compensation patterns created by fatigue, but more importantly, it can lead to injury. When training power with VBT, I look for velocity losses at less than 10 percent as the season draws nearer, while monitoring power output instead of bar speeds. Either can be monitored, however.

The following three examples are different ways I incorporate percentage of velocity loss into my programs when training for hypertrophy, power, and strength:

- Manipulation of reps
- Manipulation of sets
- Manipulation of load or intensity

I have chosen these three methods to demonstrate how monitoring percentages of velocity loss can be used to help manipulate reps, sets, or load (intensity) when training different traits. It is important to note that what is being demonstrated is the manipulation of the set and rep scheme. As a result, all three traits can be trained using all three methods.

Table 6.3 provides a summary of the three methods discussed in this section.

Table 6.3 EXAMPLES OF THREE METHODS FOR TARGETING DIFFERENT TRAINING ADAPTATIONS

	SETS	REPS	INTENSITY OR LOAD	TARGET VELOCITY LOSS	REST	TRAINING ADAPTATION
Method I	8	?	0.75-1.0 m/sec (40%-70% 1RM)	40%-50%	1 min	Muscular hypertrophy
Method II	?	3	0.75-1.0 m/sec (40%-70% 1RM)	<10%	1 min	Speed or power
Method III	8	3	0.50-0.75 m/sec (60%-80% 1RM)	10%-20%	2 min	Strength or power development

Method I: Rep Manipulation Based on Velocity Loss

I use this method when training muscular hypertrophy and muscular endurance (short). It is designed to use the same weight for a predetermined number of sets. The reps are terminated once a velocity loss of greater than 50 percent target velocity is recorded. If the athlete can move the weight at the desired velocity for more than 20 reps or beyond one minute for any given set, the load must be increased.

TARGET VELOCITY LOSS

40 to 50 percent

ADAPTATION

Muscular hypertrophy (hypertrophy I)

ENERGY SYSTEM

Lactic, aerobic

SETS AND REPS

8 sets × ? reps at 40 to 70 percent 1RM, or 0.75 to 1.0 meters per second (as long as reps do not exceed 20 or one minute total work time per set)

REST

One minute between sets

PROTOCOL

1. Select desired load and velocity (0.75 to 1.0 meters per second).
2. Load does not change; perform set until the rep target velocity drops by 40 percent. For example: If 0.80 meters per second is the target velocity, the set ends when the first rep below 40 percent target velocity (0.32 meters per second) is recorded. Note: Always provide a second chance. Many times, athletes will rise to the occasion by pushing themselves a bit harder to meet the required parameters to continue. If the athlete fails two sets in a row, either lower the weight or terminate that specific workout.
3. If athletes can move the bar at a desired velocity for more than 20 reps or longer than one minute during a set, or if they can maintain the same amount of reps for all eight sets while maintaining the required velocity loss, the bar weight is too light and needs to be increased.

Method II: Set Manipulation Based on Velocity Loss

I use this method when training for power and power endurance (covered in detail in chapter 10). Once again, it is designed to use the same weight and same repetitions throughout all working sets. The sets are terminated when an average velocity loss for a set is greater than 10 to 15 percent of the athlete's initial average for a set's target velocity is recorded. Again, always provide a second chance.

TARGET VELOCITY LOSS

Less than 10 percent

ADAPTATION

Speed or power

ENERGY SYSTEM

ATP-PC energy system (power sports)

SETS AND REPS

? sets × 3 reps at 40 to 70 percent 1RM, or 0.75 to 1.0 meters per second

REST

One minute between sets

PROTOCOL

1. Select desired load or velocity (0.75 to 1.0 meters per second).
2. Establish the first set's average velocity, which becomes your marker.
3. Continue sets until any set's average velocity drops below 10 percent of the first set. For example, if 0.80 meters per second is the target velocity, the workout is over when the first set with an average set velocity loss above 10 to 15 percent (0.68 meters per second) is recorded. Again, always provide a second chance. Note: If the athlete can complete 8 to 10 full sets with a velocity loss less than 5 percent on each set, then the load is too light and more weight needs to be added.

Method III: Load Manipulation Based on Velocity Loss

I use this method when training maximal and submaximal (accelerative) strength. This method is slightly different because it is designed to change the load from set to set if losses in velocity of 10 to 20 percent are recorded. It is also used to gauge an athlete's training readiness for that particular day. Loads are adjusted any time a velocity loss greater than 10 to 20 percent of target velocity is recorded.

TARGET VELOCITY LOSS

20 to 30 percent

ADAPTATION

Strength, force development; This is also a good method for testing daily training readiness. Load is based on the athlete's recovery on that given day.

ENERGY SYSTEM

ATP-PC (sets lasting 1 to 10 seconds), lactic (sets lasting 10 seconds to one minute)

SETS AND REPS

8 sets × 3 reps at 60 to 80 percent 1RM, or 0.50 to 0.75 meters per second

REST

Two minutes between sets

PROTOCOL

1. Select desired load or velocity (0.50 to 0.75 meters second).
2. Increase or decrease the load from set to set in order to maintain target velocity within 10 to 20 percent for all eight sets.

TESTING CNS READINESS WITH VBT

When doing daily testing, the jury is still out about which types of movements are better to gauge training readiness. Most coaches use larger movements, such as CMJ jumps, but my personal preference is to use smaller and faster movements, such as pogo jumps, for the simple reason that these movements allow less time for the athlete to compensate for fatigue than the larger ones do (see figure 6.5).

Performing jump testing before a training program begins can be used as a baseline to monitor fatigue. I like to use 10 pogo jumps for height

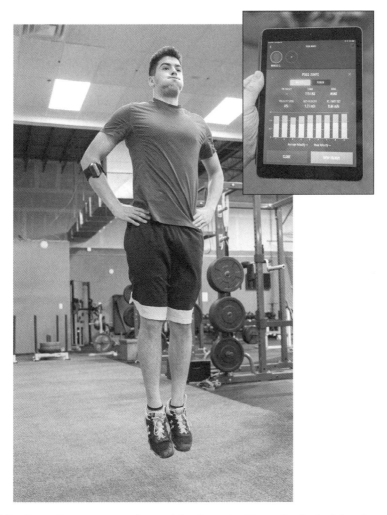

Figure 6.5   Pogo jumps are performed for jump testing prior to training to monitor fatigue.

and then take the average velocity of the set. On high-intent days, or days with a rate of perceived exertion (RPE) of nine or 10, we perform the test again and look for an average velocity that is within 10 percent of the athlete's original baseline. For anything less than 10 percent, we reduce volume by 20 percent for that day. For anything below 20 percent, we eliminate the high-intensity workout altogether. The reason for this is that the athlete's CNS is not up to the task, making the risk for injury much higher. Table 6.4 shows three different scenarios over the course of four different training days for an athlete with a baseline test of 0.92 meters per second average for pogo jumps.

As we can see on day 1, this athlete was within the 10-percent velocity loss of the original 0.92 meters per second baseline testing, so training would proceed as usual. However, on day 2, after playing a double overtime match the day before, there is enough CNS fatigue to warrant a decrease in volume of 20 percent. On day 4, multiple stressors—from game play to midterms and a lack of adequate sleep—have brought CNS fatigue considerably below the baseline, so it would be best to skip high-intensity training on this day altogether. And finally, on day 4, post-midterms and after some much-needed rest, levels are back to normal and even slightly above. Training would resume and load or volume would be increased if needed.

This example perfectly illustrates how easy it can be to train when readiness is low. Overtraining or overreaching can result from a fatigued CNS. However, with VBT, we are now able to put some tangible numbers to CNS fatigue and possibly help athletes keep recovery levels more stable throughout the training period and beyond.

Table 6.4 FOUR-DAY BASELINE AVERAGE FOR 10 POGO JUMPS FOR AN ATHLETE WITH 0.92 METERS PER SECOND BASELINE VELOCITY

DAY 1	0.84 m/sec	9% velocity loss	Ready to train
DAY 2	0.79 m/sec	14% velocity loss	Decrease volume by 20%
DAY 3	0.72 m/sec	21% velocity loss	Skip high-intensity day altogether
DAY 4	0.97 m/sec	0% velocity loss	Ready to train

I have found VBT to be a game changer for autoregulation, the process that allows coaches and athletes to adjust to these individual stressors based on velocity losses within the set or from day to day. Overall volume–load (load × reps × sets) is reduced as a result of loss and fatigue to prevent athletes from performing unnecessary repetitions and hampering the desired adaptation.

One study suggests that the cutoff velocities of 10 to 30 percent can be used to limit metabolic stress while optimizing a strength-training stimulus and limiting the hampering effects of fatigue (Pareja-Blanco et al. 2016). The same study stated that using lower percentages (around 40 to 50 percent 1RM) not only allows for higher rep sets but also creates a higher time under tension. This elicits greater muscle damage and, in turn, increases in the cross-sectional area of type I muscle fibers. In other words, as fatigue sets in, velocity slows down, and VBT helps keep us in check on all counts.

PROGRAMMING

THE USE OF FILLERS

In the following programs, exercises are numbered as 1a and 1b, 2a and 2b, and so on. For example, the "1b" exercise is a mobility exercise used as a filler incorporated into the main exercise's (1a) rest period. Fillers accomplish two things: They not only help maintain density in the program because time is usually a constraint but also account for some of the required rest periods between sets of the main lift. For example, let's suppose a deadlift is numbered as 1a. The 1b exercise that immediately follows this deadlift will be done as some sort of mobility exercise. I calculate approximately one minute of the required rest period to performing the filler exercise. So, if we were in the strength phase and required a three-minute rest, it would look something like this:

	Exercise	Sets	Reps	Rest	Tempo	VBT velocity (m/sec)
1a	Deadlift	5	3	—	Explosive	0.40-0.50
1b	Hip CARS	4	6 per side	2 min	—	—

The following chapters cover the various training blocks, or phases. The five training phases comprise a complete one-year macrocycle of training, or a yearly plan. These phases are arranged in the following chronological order: from the beginning of the preparatory period (early off-season) through the transition (transfer to sport) and competitive (in-season) periods.

It is important to note that intermittent periods of competition keep some athletes from having a full six months to train. In this case, the recommendation is to have the coach or athlete work backward, or back out, from the first day of competition and make sure that strength and the transfer of power to sport are always included.

Note: I have not included a second transition or recovery period in this text because the time (two-to-four weeks) is generally treated as a recovery period and primarily involves intervals of complete rest. Training, however, can and should be done if the athlete or coach feels that a lower volume of accelerative strength work combined with complete rest would be more beneficial than total time off to adequately recover and prepare for the next off-season plan. If this is the case, my recommendation is to use a short phase of submaximal strength (phase III) at 70 percent of the volume generally prescribed in that phase.

Since most of my work involves working with elite baseball players every day, I have provided an example of a yearly plan as it pertains to high school or college baseball athletes and their season. This could, however, be adapted to any sport and the sport's yearly timing. As mentioned previously, when looking at the different phases, keep in mind that the amount of time spent in each phase differs slightly from sport to sport and from athlete to athlete. The following table is an example of how I would lay out yearly training for a baseball player.

PERIOD	PHASE	TRAINING VOLUME	PLAYING VOLUME
Preparatory (early off-season)	Phase I: tissue prep Phase II: hypertrophy I, II	Moderate to high	Low
Preparatory (mid–off-season)	Phase III: submaximal and maximal strengths	High	Low
Transition I (late off-season to preseason)	Phase IV: power, muscular endurance	Moderate	Moderate to high
Competitive (in-season)	Phase V: strength-power maintenance	Low	High
Transition II (postseason)	Strength maintenance, recovery	Low to moderate	Low

Yearly Periodization Using VBT

The ultimate success of any training program centers on the ability to produce specific physiological adaptations that will translate into increases in performance (Poliquin 1988). This is achieved by using a concept called periodization for yearly programming. Without being familiar with a few key concepts of periodization, trying to apply bar and body speeds with VBT or any method will be premature at best. In previous chapters, we discussed in detail what VBT actually is, what its origins are, and how to read the data as well as monitor fatigue. We now turn to two of the most frequently asked questions regarding programming and the use of VBT.

1. How do I program and use VBT over a complete training year for an athlete or a team?
2. How do I break up the year's training into different phases?

To answer these questions, we must first have a discussion about periodization. We cannot effectively program for an athlete until we have reached a basic understanding of periodization. This chapter briefly explains training cycles and periods, breaking them down into various phases as well as the hierarchy (i.e., continuum) of these phases to reveal how and where the special strength zones (from chapter 4) fit into them.

PERIODIZATION: TRAINING CYCLES, PERIODS, AND PHASES

Periodization is an organized approach to training with the intent of maximizing recovery in order to elicit a performance effect. Periodization organizes a yearly or seasonal plan by partitioning it into smaller training periods and phases throughout the course of the athlete's year or season in order to maximize competitive performance.

In periodization, the structure (periods and phases) and timing (cycle) of these periods and phases highly depend on the following:

- The sport and type of athlete you are training
- The team's or athlete's specific needs
- The period or phase the team or athlete is currently in

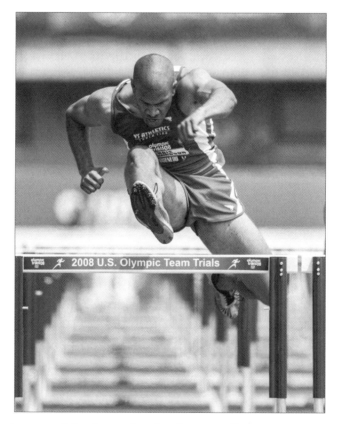

2008 U.S. Olympic Team Trials

By partitioning an athlete's yearly plan into smaller training periods, we can maximize recovery and maximize in-season performance.

© Human Kinetics

Each of these factors profoundly affects the program design and the desired training adaptation. For example, a professional baseball player has a very long season (approximately six months) that is followed by a long off-season (approximately five months). This makes programming somewhat easier to structure for a professional athlete than, say, for a high school soccer player who has multiple shorter competitive periods throughout the year.

Periodization is an organized approach to training with the intent of maximizing recovery in order to elicit a performance effect.

Once we structure the training plan, we can use VBT in our programming by simply assigning the appropriate velocity, which will allow us to use one of the five special strength zones. This will then make it possible to shift our focus to the particular adaptation that we are trying to achieve in that particular phase. The following chapters cover this in greater detail, but, for now, we will take a closer look at what cycles, periods, and phases are and how to organize them as a yearly training program specifically designed for individual athletes or teams.

Training Cycles

Training cycles (generally referred to as macrocycles, mesocycles, and microcycles) are implemented into a program as measurements of time that athletes will spend in a particular period or phase. These cycles are then broken down further into periods and phases. Table 7.1 provides the NSCA's (2016) hierarchy and parameters of these cycles.

Training cycles are implemented into a program as measurements of time that athletes will spend in a particular period or phase.

Only when we understand how and when to use cycles can we begin to structure the athlete's training program. The program usually occurs for an off-season (seasonal) or throughout the year (yearly plan).

Table 7.1 PERIODIZATION CYCLES FOR A YEARLY PLAN

TRAINING CYCLE	DURATION	DESCRIPTION
Macrocycle	Several months to one year (dependent upon schedule of the specific sport)	Generally used when timing periods or yearly plans
Mesocycle	Two to six weeks	Generally used when timing phases or blocks with the most common time frame being four to six weeks
Microcycle	Several days to two weeks	Smallest training cycle with the most common time frame being one week

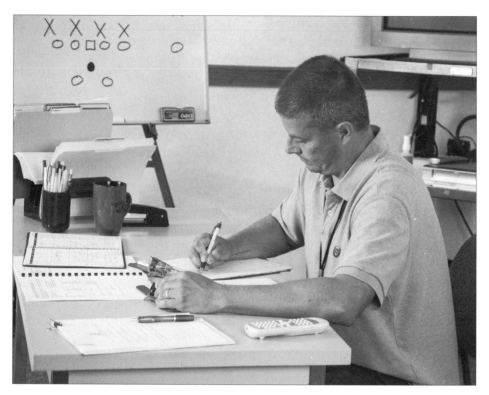

Once we understand cycles, including how and when they are used, we can then begin to structure the athlete's training program.

© Human Kinetics

Training Periods

We use the training cycles to partition the year into training periods that are put together in a continuum, which, just like the body, is dynamic and progressive in its adaptation. Therefore, the periodization and programming of these periods should also be treated as a continuum. This way we can more efficiently implement the many different phases of training used throughout an athlete's yearly plan. I break this yearly plan (macrocycle) into four different training periods, which helps me systematically organize an athlete's or a team's training with the main goal of promoting peak condition once competition (in-season) comes around.

For the scope of this text, we will use an example of a yearly plan because it includes all training periods and phases and the velocities that are associated with each type of strength. Any or all of these parameters can then be applied to the structure of any athlete's individualized training program specific to the athlete's particular sport and competitive schedule. A sample yearly plan for a baseball player would look like this:

- *Preparatory period.* This period is the early or mid–off-season and lasts approximately four to five months.
- *Transition period I (conversion to sport).* This period is the late off-season or preseason and lasts approximately 6 to 12 weeks.
- *Competitive period.* This period is the in-season and duration is dependent upon the sport.
- *Transition period II.* This period is the post-season or recovery and lasts approximately one to four weeks.

Training Phases

The training periods are then further broken down into mesocycles, or what is often referred to as training blocks or phases. (For the scope of this text, we will simply refer to them as phases.) These phases help to guide the coach or athlete to the training focus and to design a well-structured and efficient training plan whose end goal is to reach peak performance when the competitive period, or in-season, arrives.

Note that these phases are considered mesocycles because they are at least two to six weeks long. I personally rarely use microcycles (one to two weeks long) because I believe at least one week should be devoted to motor learning before we can even consider ourselves really working within that phase. Thus, I generally work in four- to six-week phases.

To specifically address all the different ways yearly and monthly plans are laid out would require a whole other text. Table 7.2 shows an example

Table 7.2 SAMPLE YEARLY TRAINING PLAN FOR BASEBALL PLAYERS

PERIOD	PREPARATORY	TRANSITION I	COMPETITIVE	TRANSITION II
SEASON	Early or mid–off-season	Late off-season or preseason	In-season	Postseason or recovery
DURATION	3-5 months	6-12 weeks	Dependent upon the sport	1-4 weeks
PHASE (FOCUS)	Tissue prep, hypertrophy I (submaximal strength), hypertrophy II (maximal strength)	Power endurance and muscular endurance	Strength and power maintenance	Maintenance of accelerative strength (strength-speed) or complete rest
SPECIAL STRENGTH ZONES USED	Strength-speed, accelerative strength, absolute strength	Strength-speed, speed-strength, absolute strength	Accelerative strength, strength-speed, speed-strength	Strength-speed and accelerative strength

of a yearly plan with the partitioning of training periods and phases that I use when working and programming for baseball players. Once again, these phases and their approximate durations can vary based on the sport, the timing of the sport, and the individual athlete.

YEARLY PROGRAMMING WITH VBT

To be able to train more efficiently with VBT, we must first expand our understanding of training periods and what we are trying to accomplish when breaking them down into phases.

Preparatory Period

The goal of the preparatory period (early or mid–off-season) is to develop a baseline of tensile strength, lean muscle mass, and absolute strength so that athletes can train at higher intensities and speeds in later phases when transitioning to sport. The preparatory period's training phases generally include the following:

- **Tissue prep** (0.75 to 1.0 meters per second)
- **Hypertrophy I** (0.75 to 1.0 meters per second)
- **Hypertrophy II** (0.40 to 0.60 meters per second)
- **Absolute strength** (<0.50 meters per second)

Core lifts such as squats, deadlifts, and bench presses and rows are the primary focus in the preparatory period. We use compound lifts (lifts that use multi-joint movements) early on to address overall strength of the prime movers while simultaneously working the accessory muscles (calves, triceps, etc.). We use heavier loads and long times under tension to create these adaptations in this period, so not much sport-specific work is done at this time.

Core lifts such as squats, deadlifts, and bench presses and rows are the primary focus in the preparatory period.

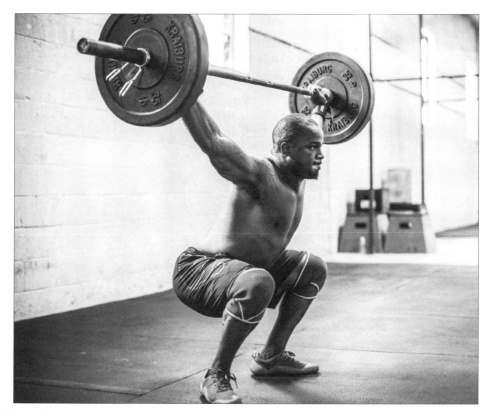

Developing a good, solid base of strength in the preparatory period helps prepare the athlete for higher intensities and speeds later in the off-season.

© MoMo Productions/Stone Sub/Getty Images

Transition Period I (Conversion to Sport)

The transition I period (late off-season or preseason) takes the strength gained in the preparatory period and works on translating it into both the strength side of power (strength–power) and speed side of power (speed-strength). Which strength to use for training these types of power takes a higher priority and depends on both the athlete and the athlete's respective sport. (This is covered in more detail in chapter 10.) The following training phases are generally used in the transition I period:

- **Absolute strength**
  (<.50 meters per second)
- **Strength-speed**
  (0.75 to 1.0 meters per second)
- **Speed-strength**
  (1.0 to 1.3 meters per second)

The adaptations previously attained earlier in the off-season training transfer over to the performance of the athlete's specific sport, and exercises, at this point, will begin to mimic movements closer to that of the athlete's sport (see figure 7.1). For example, if we were training a basketball player or wide receiver in football, exercises such as walking lunges and lateral lunges could be used for training strength-power, and loaded jumps could be used for training speed-power.

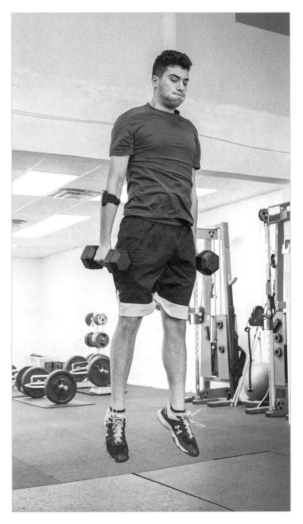

Figure 7.1   Learning to quickly apply the strength gained in the preparatory period to the athlete's respective sport is the primary focus in the first transition period.

Competitive Period

During the competitive period (in-season), we maintain or even continue to increase strength and power slightly as we decrease volume. Decreasing volume (usually sets and reps), as well as eliminating any eccentric tempos greater than 2-0-0, reduces our chances of causing any residual soreness that may translate to next day. It is also important to note the use of a conjugate style of training due to the specific training residuals that occur from playing competitive sport during this time. This is done in order to address several adaptations with little time available to train in the gym (more on this in chapter 11). The following training phases are generally used in the competitive period:

- **Accelerative strength** (0.50 to 0.75 meters per second)
- **Strength-speed** (0.75 to 1.0 meters per second)
- **Speed-strength** (1.0 to 1.3 meters per second)

Exercises and energy system work mimic movements specific to a sport and may include: core lifts such as squat variations and bench variations at 0.50 to 0.75 meters per second, or 60 to 80 percent 1RM, (accelerative strength); weighted jumps and Olympic lifts at 0.75 to 1.3 meters per second, or 20 to 60 percent 1RM, (strength-speed or speed-strength); and sprint work and change-of-direction (COD) drills (body weight to 20 percent) (see figure 7.2).

Transition Period II

Recovery is of the utmost importance in the transition II (post-season or recovery) period. This may include taking complete time off to allow the athlete to regroup both physically and mentally before beginning a new annual training plan or rehabilitating an injury. Another option is to perform a low volume of strength training to maintain strength levels while incorporating soft tissue and mobility work to expedite recovery. This option involves lighter strength training at low sets and intensities (volume), during which VBT can still be used sparingly. Unless more time is warranted for an injury, it is recommended to spend no more than one to four weeks in this period; otherwise an athlete will have to devote much more time in the following preparatory period when beginning the next macrocycle.

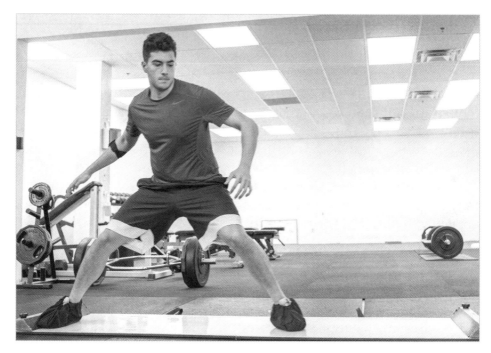

Figure 7.2 In the competitive period, exercises and energy system work that mimic those movements of the sport are the most effective choices.

LINEAR AND UNDULATING PERIODIZATION

This section covers the two most popular methods of periodization: linear and nonlinear (also known as undulating). We will first take a brief look at each and discuss when one method may be the better option of the two.

Linear Periodization

In 1964, Leon Matveyev popularized linear periodization. It typically involves staying in the same loading zone *over an entire mesocycle* before transitioning into a different loading zone or training phase. Doing so allows the athlete to stay in a particular training adaptation for a longer period of time.

Linear periodization is the most common method used with novice athletes and athletes who can afford a longer (greater than eight weeks) off-season. This type of programming is appealing because it prepares the athlete's body to accept more variations in future training. This plays a considerable role in-season because the longer we train a strength adaptation, the longer it takes before that trait begins to decline once game play starts. For example, an athlete who stays in a maximal strength phase for four to eight weeks through linear periodization will retain that strength for a longer period of time than an athlete who trained strength only one time a week for a month in a nonlinear, or undulating, model. (Chapter 11 covers this in greater detail with in-season training and training residuals.)

A linear method can be applied in two ways:

- *Sets and reps remain the same, while intensity and volume increase.* The early-to-mid–off-season is a better time for this method to be used for building strength because it produces an increase in overall volume as the phase progresses. (See table 7.3. Remember that VBT ranges are estimates.)

- *Intensity increases while training volume decreases.* This decrease in volume occurs when sets and reps are adjusted within the training phases. The late off-season is a better time to use this method when training progresses toward competition. (See table 7.4. Remember that VBT ranges are estimates.)

I use a linear method of periodization for most of my athlete's yearly plan. However, I do move to a nonlinear (undulating) method during the in-season and sometimes in the transition periods as well if practice or time becomes an issue and limits time in the weight room.

Table 7.3 LINEAR PERIODIZATION MESOCYCLE DURING A STRENGTH PHASE WHEN BOTH VOLUME AND INTENSITY INCREASE

WEEK 1	WEEKS 2 AND 3	WEEK 4
5 × 5 sets or reps at 0.65-0.75 m/sec (60% 1RM)	5 × 5 sets or reps at 0.60-0.70 m/sec (70% 1RM)	5 × 5 sets or reps at 0.50-0.60 m/sec (80% 1RM)

Table 7.4 LINEAR PERIODIZATION MESOCYCLE DURING A POWER PHASE WHEN VOLUME DECREASES AND INTENSITY INCREASES

WEEK 1	WEEKS 2 AND 3	WEEK 4
8 × 2 sets or reps at 0.65-0.75 m/sec (60% 1RM)	6 × 2 sets or reps at 0.60-0.70 m/sec (70% 1RM)	4 × 2 sets or reps at 0.50-0.60 m/sec (80% 1RM)

Nonlinear, or Undulating, Periodization

In 1988, Charles Poliquin popularized nonlinear, or undulating, periodization, the method that involves weekly or daily fluctuations in both training load and volume and trains different adaptations within a particular time period. Nonlinear periodization does not provide a long enough saturation period of anatomical adaptation (phases) in the early and mid–off-seasons because we are training different traits weekly or even daily during this time. However, the appeal is the ability to focus on multiple training adaptations (phases) at one time whether they are daily, weekly, or biweekly (microcycle), which allows the athlete's body to respond to a variety of challenges within a weekly program (unlike a more linear model that only focuses on one strength trait at a time). As a result, nonlinear periodization is ideal for in-season programming in order for athletes to maintain several different qualities while playing their sport (see table 7.5). This, too, is covered in more detail in chapter 11. Nonlinear periodization is the time during the year when I employ the use of microcycles.

Table 7.5 UNDULATING PERIODIZATION MICROCYCLE WHEN TRAINING DIFFERENT ADAPTATIONS WITHIN THE SAME WEEK

MONDAY	WEDNESDAY	FRIDAY
5 × 5 sets or reps at 0.50-0.60 m/sec, or 80% 1RM (maximal strength)	6 × 3 sets or reps at 0.80-0.90 m/sec, or 50% 1RM (strength-power)	8 × 3 sets or reps at 0.90-1.0 m/sec, or 40% 1RM (speed-power)

The amount of time and effort, the type of work and, most importantly, the time frame during which training occurs shapes and determines an athlete's conditioning level. This is why programming with VBT is advantageous for a coach or an athlete. However, much like traditional percentage-based training, finding a system that works for you and your athletes requires a lot of trial and error: The more you use VBT in your programming, the more efficient you will get at using it. All of the information I have provided is from my own research and personal experiences. I recommend this as a good place for you to start, but, like anything, let the numbers talk to you and help you draw your own conclusions from the data. This is the best way to ensure that VBT will work for you and your specific clients.

Early Off-Season: Tissue Prep and Hypertrophy

After a long season and only a few weeks of recovery, many athletes will still need to pay extra care to their joints going into the next early off-season. Once again, assessing your athlete's current conditioning level is of paramount importance to determine where to begin from both a mobility and a strength standpoint. This is where VBT excels in giving the athlete and coach alike external information about appropriate velocity levels for gauging volume and autoregulation for keeping in perspective an athlete's week-to-week and day-to-day recovery status.

It is important to note that these programs are only starting points, meaning that there is no perfect program that works for every athlete. Remember, much is predicated upon the following:

- The needs of the sport (e.g., biomechanical profile, common injury sites, position-specific)
- An athlete's current conditioning level (e.g., movement screen, strength testing injury history)

It is important to keep in mind that many athletes expect to see huge leaps in performance after only four to six weeks of strength training. However, athletes generally do not experience the highest peaks in performance until the competitive period, or at best, when the competitive period draws near. Strength, much like athletic ability and technique, is a skill that can be developed much the same way through various methods and phases. These phases begin with the off-season and progress toward a peak at the beginning of the competitive period (in-season).

The two primary phases in the early off-season are phase I tissue prep and phase II hypertrophy, and their primary goal is to prepare the athlete in both strength and conditioning for heavier lifting later in the off-season.

Phase I: Tissue Prep

Phase I tissue prep is the foundation for the other phases of training, and knowing this is especially crucial before entering into a strength phase where volume and load are higher. I have found that athletes who skip phase I and jump right into phase II hypertrophy do not reap the same benefits in later phases as those athletes who spend the necessary four to six weeks in this phase first. The name of this phase reflects the fact that the main objective is not to achieve an immediate overload, but, rather, to elicit a progressive adaptation of the athlete's anatomy and tensile strength. While this phase does not focus on hypertrophy specifically, increases in cross-sectional area may develop due to the isometric time under tension nature of the training. In addition, an extended amount of time is spent in the eccentric and isometric phases of the exercise (see figure 8.1).

GOALS

The main goals during the tissue-prep phase are the following:

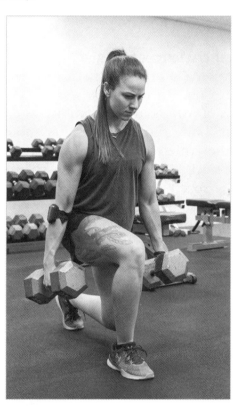

- *Improving tensile strength.* This phase prepares the tendons, ligaments, and joints for longer, more strenuous sessions in later phases. This is partially because hydrogen ions, which are released by lactic acid, have been proven to stimulate the release of growth hormone and, therefore, collagen synthesis (5). Using isometric holds in low positions increases time under tension and solidifies movement patterns where they are at the biggest mechanical disadvantage. Both tissue-prep and hypertrophy phases help increase applications of force in later phases when heavier loads are being used.

Figure 8.1 In a tissue-prep phase, using isometric holds in low positions increases time under tension, as well as solidifying movement patterns where they are at the biggest mechanical disadvantage.

- *Regrooving good movement patterns.* This involves multiple muscle groups in order to groove or re-groove more efficient motor patterns (neuromuscular coordination) specific to the athlete's sport. For this reason, longer eccentric tempos and isometric holds are implemented using low-resistance loads. However, concentric phases should remain explosive to stimulate fast-twitch fibers.

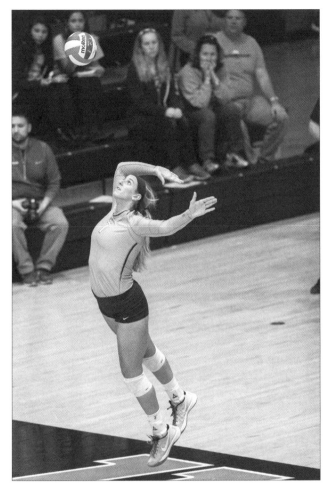

All sports involve explosive movements. For this reason, even when longer eccentric tempos and isometric holds are implemented in a tissue-prep phase, concentric tempos should remain explosive to stimulate type II (fast-twitch) fibers.

© Human Kinetics

TRAINING PARAMETERS

Types of exercises	Multi-joint exercises such as squats, deadlifts, bench presses, rowing exercises, push-ups, and chin-ups should be used to better stimulate the release of anabolic hormones, promoting muscle growth while strengthening the prime movers used in sport activities. Isolation exercises such as biceps curls and triceps extensions should be kept to a minimum.	
Training intensity	The duration of time under tension is long, so low intensities as well as high-velocity losses are used in both the tissue-prep phase and phase II for hypertrophy I.	40%-60% 1RM (increasing weekly)

VBT velocity	Start all athletes at 1.0 m/sec, and increase intensity weekly to 0.75-0.80 m/sec based on the desired percentage of 1RM. Note: *Because these first two phases involve maximum fatigue, VBT velocities are used only to provide a starting point. VBT is primarily used in these first two phases to monitor velocity loss to gauge reps and time.*	0.75-1.0 m/sec (starting velocity only)
VBT velocity loss	30%-40%	
Tempo	Eccentric and isometric training are emphasized to maintain conditioning of the type II fibers. Concentric phases are still performed explosively.	3-1-0, 3-2-0, 4-2-0
Reps	Start all athletes at 12-15 reps, and decrease weekly down to 6-8 reps. Time under tension should vary anywhere between 40-70 seconds. This time under tension involves the anaerobic lactic system as the main energy system. (See chapter 6, Method II: Set Manipulation Based On Velocity Loss section.)	12-15 down to 8 reps (decreasing weekly by 2 reps, and incorporating velocity loss into rep scheme)
Sets	2-4 per exercise	
Rest	1-2 min between sets	
Frequency of training	2-4 sessions per week (full body: 2-3 per week; splits: 4 per week [2 upper, 2 lower])	

PROGRAMMING

SAMPLE LOWER-BODY PROGRAM FOR DAYS 1 AND 3

Warm-up		EXERCISE	SETS	TIME	REST	TEMPO	VBT VELOCITY (M/SEC)
	1	Tempo runs	1	30 sec	30 sec	—	—

Power plyometrics		EXERCISE	SETS	REPS	REST	TEMPO	VBT VELOCITY (M/SEC)
	1a	Pogo jump	3	20	—	As fast as possible	—
	1b	90-90 hip flexor with band serratus	2	5	1 min	—	—
	2a	Seated box jump	3	5	—	Explosive	—
	2b	Wall dribbles	2	20	—		

Main		EXERCISE	SETS	REPS	REST	TEMPO	VBT VELOCITY (M/SEC)
	1a	Trap bar deadlift	3	12	—	3-2-0	0.75-1.0
	1b	Hip-flow circuit	3	2 per side	1 min	—	—
	2a	Back squat	3	12	—	3-2-0	0.75-1.0
	2b	Dead bug	3	8 per side	1 min	—	—
	3a	Lateral slide board lunge	3	8 per side	—	—	—
	3b	Half-kneeling cable chop	3	8 per side	1 min	—	—

SAMPLE UPPER-BODY PROGRAM FOR DAYS 2 AND 4

Warm-up		EXERCISE	SETS	TIME	REST	TEMPO	VBT VELOCITY (M/SEC)
	1	Airdyne bike	1	5 min	—	—	—

Power plyometrics		EXERCISE	SETS	REPS, TIME	REST	TEMPO	VBT VELOCITY (M/SEC)
	1a	Plyo chest press	3	20 reps	—	As fast as possible	—
	1b	Straight-leg hip turns	3	5 reps per side	1 min	—	—
	2a	Split stance recoil slams	3	6 reps per side	—	Explosive	—
	2b	Bear crawl	3	30 sec	1 min	—	—

Main		EXERCISE	SETS	REPS, TIME	REST	TEMPO	VBT VELOCITY (M/SEC)
	1a	One-arm cable row	3	12 reps per side	—	3-2-0	—
	1b	Side-lying external rotation	3	10 reps	—	—	—
	1c	Wall press abs	3	8 reps per side	1 min	—	—
	2a	Bench press	3	12 reps	—	3-2-0	—
	2b	Side plank	3	6 10-sec reps per side	1 min	—	—
	2c	Half kneeling cable chop	3	8 reps per side	—	—	—
	3a	Suspension row	3	12 reps	—	3-2-0	—
	3b	Medicine ball halo	3	5 reps per side	1 min	—	—

Note: It is important to remember to maintain explosiveness in the concentric portion of the lift by using VBT in this and all phases. This helps maintain fast-twitch type II fibers while type I fibers are the focus.

Phase II: Hypertrophy

Once a good base of tensile strength has been developed in phase I, it is time for the athlete to work on increasing the lean body mass in phase II that will be translated into increased functional performance in later phases. To achieve this, an athlete increases not only the mechanical stress to the muscle fibers but also the load used, the total time under tension (especially of the eccentric phase), and the total volume of sets and reps—in other words, hypertrophy. The main difference between the two types, hypertrophy I and hypertrophy II, is motor unit recruitment (see figure 8.2). Each muscle contains a series of differently sized fibers: the low-threshold, or smaller, weaker fibers and the high-threshold, or larger, stronger fibers.

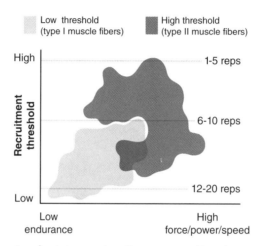

Figure 8.2 In hypertrophy I, increasing the cross-sectional area of the low-threshold fibers involves using lower intensities with higher reps. But, as load intensity increases in hypertrophy II, high-threshold motor units are recruited earlier.

Hypertrophy I

This phase involves performing resistance training and focusing on increasing low-threshold muscle fibers in the cross-sectional area. These fibers are recruited during the first few reps of a set, and then the high-threshold fibers are recruited sequentially as needed when the athlete gets closer to failure. Using lighter loads and longer time under tension make hypertrophy I very effective in the early phases of the off-season for athletes whose main focus is to maximize lean muscle mass. Hypertrophy I is also used in bodybuilding for achieving aesthetic size and muscle symmetry; this phase is centered around an increase in the type I slow-twitch muscle fiber.

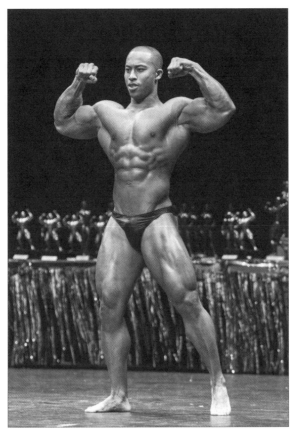

While hypertrophy I is the main training adaptation used in bodybuilding, it is also useful in early phases of training for athletic performance.

© Human Kinetics

TRAINING PARAMETERS

Types of exercises	Multi-joint exercises such as squats, deadlifts, bench presses, rowing exercises, push-ups, and chin-ups should be used to better stimulate the release of anabolic hormones, promoting muscle growth while strengthening the prime movers used in sports. Isolation exercises should be kept to a minimum.	
Training intensity	Start all athletes at 40% 1RM or one that allows 15 reps, and increase intensity weekly by 5% until 60% is achieved or training block is completed.	40%-60% 1RM (increase weekly)
VBT velocity	Start all athletes at 1.0 m/sec, and increase intensity weekly to 0.75 m/sec based on desired percentage of 1RM. Note: Similar to phase I, the hypertrophy phase involves maximum fatigue; as a result, VBT velocities are used only to give us a starting point and are used primarily in these first two phases to monitor velocity loss to help gauge reps and time.	0.75-1.0 m/sec (starting velocities only)

VBT velocity loss	40%-50%	
Tempo	Because the neuromuscular system adapts to slow concentric movement, it does not stimulate the recruitment of fast-twitch muscle fibers that are crucial for speed- and power-dominant sports if a slow concentric movement is used. As a result, velocities are used only as a starting point in this phase. There is no need to calculate reps because the goal is to do a high number of reps to create maximum fatigue. It is important to cue athletes to always try to move the weight as fast as possible during the concentric phase of the lift.	3-0-0, 4-0-0
Reps	Start all athletes at 15-16 reps, and decrease weekly by 2 reps down to 10. Once again, this is when we are looking for higher drop-offs of 40%-50% from rep to rep or from set to set to elicit greater muscle breakdown and to optimize increases in the cross-sectional area of the type I muscle fibers.	16 down to 10 (decrease weekly by 2 reps; incorporate velocity loss into rep scheme)
Sets	3-5 sets per exercise for 10-12 total when using upper- and lower-splits, and 20-24 total when using full-body workouts	3-5 sets per exercise
Rest	The amount of rest is dependent upon the athlete's muscular endurance, which is being built up at the same time. Use the minimum amount of rest needed to hit the desired velocities prescribed, but, as intensities increase and the athlete moves closer to phase III, rest intervals should increase.	1-3 min
Frequency of training	Training should be done 2 times per week if full-body workouts are prescribed, or 4 times per week if using upper- and lower-splits.	

PROGRAMMING

SAMPLE LOWER-BODY PROGRAM FOR DAYS 1 AND 3

Warm-up		EXERCISE	SETS	TIME	REST	TEMPO	VBT VELOCITY (M/SEC)
	1	Tempo runs	5	30 sec	30 sec	—	—
Power plyometrics		EXERCISE	SETS	REPS, TIME	REST	TEMPO	VBT VELOCITY (M/SEC)
	1a	Squat jump	3	5 reps	—	Explosive	—
	1b	Hip-flow circuit	2	2 reps per side	—	—	—
	1c	Half-kneeling side starts	3	2 reps per side	—	Explosive	—
	1d	Shoulder tube	2	30 sec	1 min	—	—

Main (keep intensity between 40%-60% 1RM and velocity loss at 40%-50%)		EXERCISE	SETS	REPS, TIME	REST	TEMPO	VBT VELOCITY (M/SEC)
	1a	Barbell Romanian deadlift	5	12 reps	—	4-0-0	0.75-1.0
	1b	Yoga plex	3	30 sec	2 min	—	—
	2a	Barbell front squat	5	12 reps	—	4-0-0	0.75-1.0
	2b	Reach, roll, and lift	3	5 reps	2 min	—	—
	3a	Lateral slide board lunge	5	12 reps per side	—	4-0-0	0.75-1.0
	3b	Band distractions with perturbations	3	3 reps	2 min	—	—
Core and rotator cuff		EXERCISE	SETS	REPS, TIME	REST	TEMPO	VBT VELOCITY (M/SEC)
	1a	Plank	3	30 sec	—	—	—
	1b	Side bridge	3	8 reps per side	1 min	—	—

SAMPLE UPPER-BODY PROGRAM FOR DAYS 2 AND 4

Warm-up		EXERCISE	SETS	REPS, TIME, DISTANCE	REST	TEMPO	VBT VELOCITY (M/SEC)
	1	Airdyne bike	1	5 min			
Power plyometrics		EXERCISE	SETS	REPS	REST	TEMPO	VBT VELOCITY (M/SEC)
	1a	Medicine ball slam (8-10 lb) (4-5 kg)	3	8	—	Explosive	—
	1b	Pogo jump	2	20	1 min	As fast as possible	—
	2a	Medicine ball shovel pass (6-8 lb) (3-4 kg)	3	6 per side	—	Explosive	—
	2b	Deep-squat breathing	2	5	—	—	—

Main (keep intensity between 40%-60% 1RM and velocity loss at 40%-50%)		EXERCISE	SETS	REPS	REST	TEMPO	VBT VELOCITY (M/SEC)
	1a	Incline T-row	5	12	—	4-0-0	0.70-0.80 (starting velocity only)
	1b	Dowel trap raise	3	8	2 min		
	2a	One-arm dumbbell bench press	5	12 per side	—	4-0-0	0.70-0.80 (starting velocity only)
	2b	Bench T-spine mobility	3	5	2 min	—	—
	3a	One-arm cable row	5	12 per side	—	4-0-0	0.70-0.80 (starting velocity only)
	3b	Dead bug	3	8 per side	2 min	—	—

Core and rotator cuff		EXERCISE	SETS	REPS, DISTANCE	REST	TEMPO	VBT VELOCITY (M/SEC)
	1a	Pallof press	2	8 reps per side	—	—	—
	1b	Bear crawl	2	20 yd each way	1 min	—	—

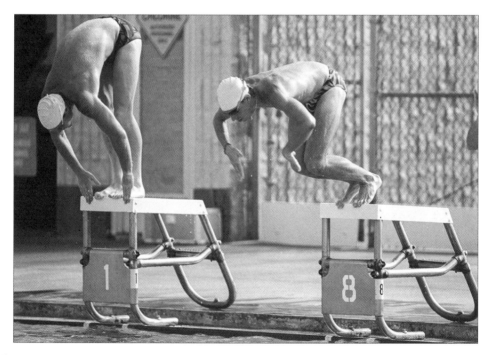

For athletes who already possess a good amount of lean muscle mass, time may be better spent in hypertrophy II in order to train faster, more efficient motor unit recruitment rather than focusing on increases in low-threshold fiber size as with hypertrophy I.

© Photodisc/Getty Images

Hypertrophy II

The focus in hypertrophy II is motor unit recruitment of the high-threshold fibers closer to the start of the lift. This is of great importance in athletic performance because we ultimately want to reduce the amount of time it takes to kick in the high-threshold motor units when playing our sport otherwise known as intramuscular coordination (see figure 8.3). This is why this type of hypertrophy is often defined as sport-specific hypertrophy.

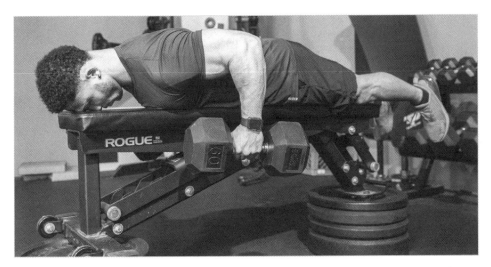

Figure 8.3 The use of exercises such as prone bench rows during a hypertrophy II phase helps better stimulate the release of anabolic hormones and increase contractile properties of high-threshold muscle fibers.

During hypertrophy II, the sizes of the specific prime movers increase without neglecting the neural component of force expression (7). This holds true for most sports, but it is especially true in high-explosive sports such as football, baseball, sprinting, and shot put and discus. Intensities used in hypertrophy II are generally higher than those in hypertrophy I, but the number of reps is lower while the set number and work–rest ratios increase. So, athletes who already possess a good amount of lean muscle mass can use hypertrophy II in place of hypertrophy I to improve motor unit recruitment. With its use of heavier loads, hypertrophy II transitions well into submaximal strength in phase III.

TRAINING PARAMETERS

Types of exercises	Multi-joint exercises such as squats, deadlifts, bench presses, rowing exercises, push-ups, and chin-ups should be used to better stimulate the release of anabolic hormones, promoting muscle growth while strengthening the prime movers used in sports. Isolation exercises should be kept to a minimum.	
Intensity	Start all athletes at 70% 1RM or one that allows 10-12 reps, and increase intensity weekly by 5% until 85% is achieved or training block is completed.	75%-85% 1RM (increase weekly)
VBT velocity	Start all athletes at 0.60-0.40 m/sec, and increase intensity weekly to 0.50 m/sec based on desired percentage of 1RM. Similar to phase I, the hypertrophy phase involves muscle fatigue; as a result, VBT velocities are used only to give us a starting point and are used primarily in these first two phases to monitor velocity loss to help gauge reps and time.	0.60-0.40 m/sec (starting velocities only)
VBT velocity loss	Once again, velocities are used only as a starting point in this phase. Because velocity losses only fall between 10%-20%, hypertrophy II is sometimes referred to as "high-load power." It is also important to cue athletes to try to move the weight as fast as possible during the concentric phase of the lift.	10%-20%
Tempo	Because hypertrophy II uses higher loads (75%-85% 1RM) to quickly recruit high-threshold muscle fibers, longer eccentric tempos are not used. Thus, standard controlled tempos of 1-0-0 or 2-0-0 are used. Hypertrophy II allows the type II fibers to remain under tension for the majority of the movement or set, resulting in hypertrophy of the these fast-twitch fibers, which differentiates this method from hypertrophy I.	1-0-0, 2-0-0
Reps	Start all athletes at 10 reps, and decrease weekly by 2 reps down to 5. Once again, this is when we are looking for velocity drop-offs of 10%-20% from rep to rep or from set to set to begin eliciting greater strength gains while optimizing increases in the cross-sectional area of the type I muscle fibers.	10 down to 5 (decrease weekly by 2 reps; incorporate velocity loss into rep scheme)
Sets	3-8 sets per exercise when using upper- and lower-splits and 20-24 total when using full-body workouts	3-8 per exercise
Rest	The amount of rest is dependent upon the athlete's muscular endurance, which is being built up at the same time. Use the minimum amount of rest needed to hit the desired velocities prescribed, but do not exceed 2-5 minutes. As intensities increase and the athlete moves closer to phase III, increase rest intervals closer to 4-5 minutes.	2-5 min
Frequency of training	Training should be done 2-3 times per week if full-body workouts are prescribed or 4 times per week if using upper- and lower-splits.	

PROGRAMMING

SAMPLE FULL-BODY PROGRAM

Warm-up		EXERCISE	SETS	TIME	REST	TEMPO	VBT VELOCITY (M/SEC)
	1	Spin bike or Airdyne bike	1	5 min	—	—	—
Power plyometrics		EXERCISE	SETS	REPS, TIME	REST	TEMPO	VBT VELOCITY (M/SEC)
	1a	Medicine ball slam (8-10 lb) (4-5 kg)	3	8 reps	1 min	—	—
	1b	Band lateral stretch	2	30 sec per side	—	—	—
	2a	Box jump	3	6 reps	—	—	—
	2b	T-spine rotation	2	8 reps per side	1 min	—	—
Main (keep intensity between 75%-85% 1RM and velocity loss at 10%-20%)		EXERCISE	SETS	REPS, TIME	REST	TEMPO	VBT VELOCITY (M/SEC)
	1a	Straight-bar deadlift	5	5-8 reps	—	2-0-0	0.50-0.60
	1b	Band hamstring stretch	4	30 sec	2 min	—	—
	2a	One-arm dumbbell row	5	5-8 reps per side	—	2-0-0	0.40-0.50
	2b	Cat-camel stretch	4	10 reps	2 min	—	—
	3a	Barbell front squat	5	5-8 reps	—	2-0-0	0.50-0.60
	3b	Sumo stretch	4	30 sec	2 min	—	—
	4a	Loaded push-up	5	5-8 reps	—	2-0-0	0.40-0.50
	4b	Doorway pectoral stretch	4	30 sec	2 min	—	—
Core		EXERCISE	SETS	REPS, TIME	REST	TEMPO	VBT VELOCITY (M/SEC)
	1a	Plank	3	30 sec	—	—	—
	1b	Side plank	3	8 reps per side	1 min	—	—

After a long season and some well-deserved time off, beginning a new preparatory period must involve getting back good form. To accomplish this, an athlete must regroove efficient movement patterns and increase both quality and strength of the tissues and tendons through tissue-prep (phase I). Further increases in lean body mass and mechanical tension for low- and high-threshold muscle fibers must then be the focus in phase II hypertrophy. This helps the athlete become better prepared for heavier loads in the upcoming phases.

Mid–Off-Season: Submaximal and Maximal Strengths

In the latter portion of the preparatory period (mid–off-season), after some time has been spent preparing the tissue ligaments and joints in phase I, as well as increasing the cross-sectional area of the muscle fibers (size) in phase II, it's time to create greater strength adaptations in phase III.

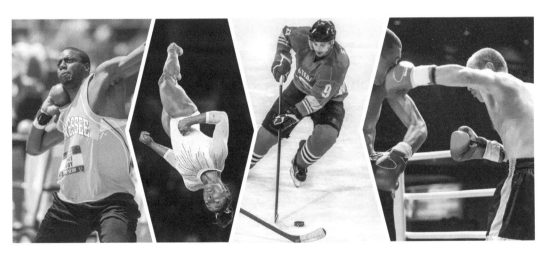

In most sports, the development of maximum strength is crucial to recruiting fast-twitch muscle fibers, their frequency of activation, and the ability to simultaneously call into action all the primary muscles involved in a given movement.

(a) © Human Kinetics; *(b)* Ulrik Pedersen/NurPhoto via Getty Images; *(c)* © vm/E+/Getty Images; *(d)* © Human Kinetics

When building out an athlete's off-season program, while all phases are important, I believe the key role is increasing general strength to its maximum because this is the foundation upon which to build all the other types of strength. In most sports, the development of maximum strength is used to recruit fast-twitch muscle fibers, their frequency of activation, and the ability to simultaneously call into action all the primary muscles involved in a given movement (Howard et al. 1985). A good example of this is during the late off-season when training power. Power is a product of strength and speed, so improving power requires improving maximum strength first. As a result, strength training is a prerequisite for attaining faster power improvement and allowing athletes to achieve higher levels of performance.

When training strength, it is important to realize that not all strength is created equal. One strength just does not work as efficiently without the other, so it is important to understand the two different categories of strength and how and when they are used:

- *General strength.* General strength is the foundation upon which all other types of strength are built, and it provides a base for the more sport-specific strength that follows. General strength is the focus of the first three phases of the off-season training plan for a more elite athlete with a higher training age (more than three years). But, for more inexperienced or novice lifters, it should be the main focus for most of the yearly plan. Intensities range from 60 to 80 percent 1RM for submaximal strength and over 80 percent 1RM for maximum strength. (Note: Spending an inadequate amount of time on general strength will negatively affect all of the future phases designed to develop sport-specific skills. Neglecting to sufficiently train this foundation can also compromise the athlete's ability to accept force, thus increasing the risk of injury.

- *Specific strength.* Specific strength training (covered in chapter 10) is incorporated into the late off-season when transferring strength gains to power or sport. Specific strength training accounts for characteristics specific to the sport regarding movement, energy system contributions, and exercises designed for continual improvement to the joints' range of motion. This training is used only after the athlete has developed an adequate level of general strength, which usually takes anywhere from one to three years. Note: Some athletes may develop general strength more quickly than others because of their genetic makeup.

To train specific strength, I use training intensities from 40 to 60 percent 1RM (0.75 to 1.0 meters per second). While heavier loads above 60 percent can still be used in the same program to train contractile properties, the majority of the program is built around the use of these lighter loads for training more sport-specific movements. Exercise selection should be based on the sport of the athlete being trained. Some examples may be hang cleans for a volleyball player, heavy sled pushes for an offensive lineman in American football, or landmine presses for a shot putter or other throwing athlete (see figure 9.1).

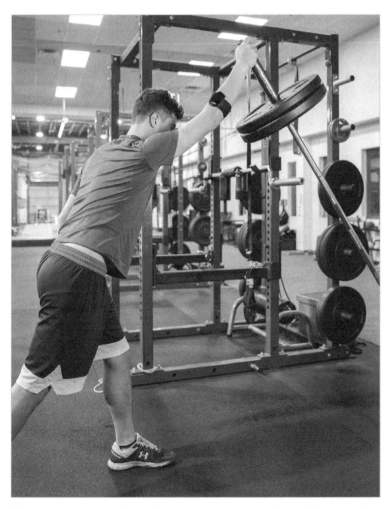

Figure 9.1 Strength training that is more specific to the sport is the focus in the late off-season, such as a shot put athlete performing landmine presses.

Phase III: Submaximal and Maximal Strengths

After building tensile strength and hypertrophy in the first two phases, phase III submaximum and maximum strength sets the foundation for all other phases that follow. This phase is slightly longer than earlier phases and comprises two three-to-four–week mesocycles, using two separate loads that start with submaximal strength and are followed by maximum strength.

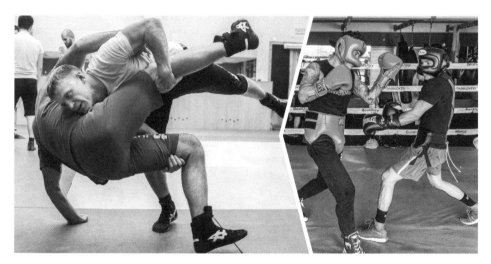

Improvements in relative strength are especially important in sports such as boxing and wrestling that involve weight classes.

(a) Valery Sharifulin\TASS via Getty Images; *(b)* Rodolfo Flores / Eyepix Group/Barcroft Media via Getty Images

GOALS

The main goals during the submaximum and maximum strength phase are the following:

- *Higher voluntary motor unit recruitment of the fast-twitch muscle fibers.* By using higher intensities and loads during a maximum strength phase, athletes are able to produce higher and more efficient recruitment of the fast-twitch fibers (see figure 9.2). This is a determinant factor in increasing power, which makes training absolute strength crucial for enabling athletes to reach a high neural output for speed- and power-dominated sports.

- *Improvements in testosterone levels and relative strength.* Increased testosterone levels help to improve maximum strength, which, in turn, helps to advance relative strength, the ratio of absolute strength to body weight. Testosterone levels in the blood increase only when the total volume of strength

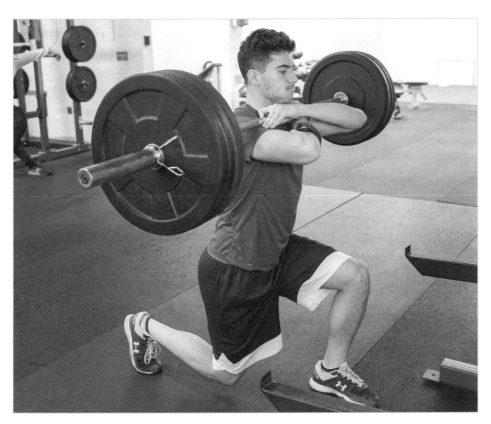

Figure 9.2 Big, multi-joint exercises involving the prime movers are the focus when training maximum strength.

training is adequate. This can vary from athlete to athlete, but levels go up generally two to three times per week. On the other hand, training absolute strength too frequently can have the opposite effect—lowering testosterone levels in the blood. This is one reason we start training maximum strength using submaximal velocities or loads.

When training in phase III, we train submaximal strength first to focus on intermuscular coordination, which involves using velocities in the accelerated strength zone. After spending a sufficient amount of time in accelerative strength (the amount of time is dependent upon the athlete), only then should training maximal strength (absolute strength) begin. Because we are training higher motor recruitment, this part of phase III involves using higher loads with velocities in the absolute strength zone, switching the training focus to intramuscular coordination. The amount of time spent in either submaximal or maximal strength varies between sports. It predominantly depends on which of these two main neural adaptations needs to be addressed more:

- *Intermuscular coordination.* This is the ability to coordinate all muscles in the kinetic chain in a single action. The goal is coordination, so core compound lifts such as deadlifts, squats, and bench presses are used in a lower submaximal strength zone (accelerative strength: 0.50 to 0.75 meters per second, or 60 to 80 percent 1RM).

- *Intramuscular coordination.* This is the capacity to recruit as many motor units as possible in the shortest amount of time. The goal is motor unit recruitment, so core compound lifts such as deadlifts, squats, and bench presses are still used, but in a higher maximum strength zone (absolute strength: less than 0.50 meters per second, or above 80% percent 1RM).

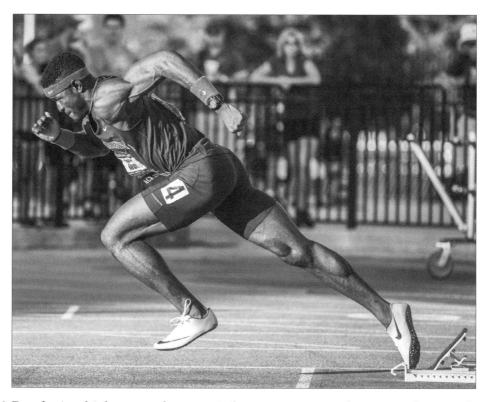

Developing higher neural output is key to activating the type II fast-twitch fibers that are vital to quick explosive sports such as sprinting.

Matt Marriott/NCAA Photos via Getty Images

TRAINING PARAMETERS

Types of exercises	Multi-joint exercises such as squats, deadlifts, and bench presses		
Training intensity	Creating the highest possible tension in the muscle is the only way to develop maximum strength. I choose to spend a longer period of time in this phase (6-8 weeks) because this phase involves the use of both moderately heavy (submaximal) and heavy (maximal) loads, *applied in this order.*	Submaximal (accelerative strength) While using maximal loads can have a higher effect on the CNS and fast-twitch fiber recruitment, it still allows for strength adaptations, but due to the lighter load, intermuscular coordination is more of a focus. Also, the combination of slightly higher velocities and slightly lower loads creates higher force output than they do in absolute strength ranges. In fact, many athletes produce the highest amount of force output in these lower ranges.	0.50-0.75 m/sec (60%-80% 1RM)
		Maximal (absolute strength) Using high loads with fewer reps causes a significant CNS adaptation: better intramuscular coordination of the muscles, resulting in an increased capacity to recruit fast-twitch fibers. Note: Both submaximal and maximal methods are percentage-based, meaning that the load indicated is a percentage of the 1RM. For this reason, before beginning phase III, *a force–velocity profile must be tested in order to accurately calculate the VBT velocities that correlate with a 1RM for the main exercises.*	<0.50 m/sec (80%-95% 1RM)
VBT velocity*	Training maximal strength requires a high demand on the CNS, so high-volume training days should never be performed under conditions of fatigue. This is another example of when VBT can engage intensity levels on high-volume days (see chapter 6).	Submaximal (accelerative strength)	0.50-.075 m/sec (60%-80% 1RM)
		Maximal (absolute strength)	<0.50 m/sec (80%-95% 1RM) (concentric phase only)
VBT velocity loss	Submaximal (accelerative strength)		20%-30%
	Maximal (absolute strength)		20%-30%
Tempo	Submaximal (accelerative strength)		2-0-0
	Maximal (absolute strength)		2-0-0

Reps	Submaximal (accelerative strength)		3-10
	Maximal (absolute strength)		1-6
Sets	Submaximal (accelerative strength)		3-8
	Maximal (absolute strength)		3-8
Rest	Rest intervals should be calculated to provide adequate recovery to the neuromuscular system and are primarily based on the athlete's fitness level.	Submaximal (accelerative strength)	2-3 min
		Maximal (absolute strength)	3-5 min
Frequency of training	Submaximal (accelerative strength)		3-4 times per week for upper- and lower-splits and 2-3 times per week for full-body workout
	Maximal (absolute strength)		3-4 times per week for upper- and lower-splits and 2-3 times per week for full-body workout

*While other methods can be used in a strength phase, such as eccentric overload and isometric training, these go beyond the scope of this text and do not require the use of VBT.

PROGRAMMING

SAMPLE SUBMAXIMAL STRENGTH (ACCELERATIVE STRENGTH) LOWER-BODY PROGRAM FOR DAYS 1 AND 3

Warm-up		EXERCISE	SETS	TIME	REST	TEMPO	VBT VELOCITY (M/SEC)
	1	Jump rope	1	5 min	—	—	—

Power plyometrics		EXERCISE	SETS	REPS, TIME	REST	TEMPO	VBT VELOCITY (M/SEC)
	1a	Medial-lateral line hop	3	12 reps per side	—	Explosive	—
	1b	Deep-squat breathing	2	30 sec	—	—	—
	2a	45-degree bounds	3	5 reps per side	—	Explosive	
	2b	Half-kneeling, shoulder-controlled articular rotation	2	5 reps per side	1 min	—	—

Main (keep intensity between 60%-80% 1RM and velocity loss at 20%-30%)		EXERCISE	SETS	REPS, DISTANCE	REST	TEMPO	VBT VELOCITY (M/SEC)
	1a	Trap bar deadlift	5	3 reps	—	Explosive	0.50-0.60
	1b	Plank with reach	3	5 reps per side	—	—	—
	1c	Half getup	3	8 reps	2 min	—	—
	2a	Split squat	5	5 reps per side	—	Explosive	0.60-0.70
	2b	Medial-lateral line hop	3	12 reps per side	—	—	—
	2c	Half-kneeling cable lift	3	8 reps per side	2 min	—	—
	3a	Single leg deadlift	4	5 reps per side	—	—	0.60-0.70
	3b	Waiter's walk	2	20 yd (18 m) per direction	2 min	—	—

SAMPLE SUBMAXIMAL STRENGTH (ACCELERATIVE STRENGTH) UPPER-BODY PROGRAM FOR DAYS 2 AND 4

Warm-up		EXERCISE	SETS	TIME	REST	TEMPO	VBT VELOCITY (M/SEC)
	1	Airdyne bike	1	5 min	—	—	—
Power plyometrics		EXERCISE	SETS	REPS, TIME	REST	TEMPO	VBT VELOCITY (M/SEC)
	1a	Plyo chest pass	3	8 reps	—	Explosive	—
	1b	90-90 hip flexor with band serratus	3	5 reps	—	—	—
	2a	Split stance overhead throw	3	6 reps	—	Explosive	—
	2b	Prone hip rotator stretch	3	30 sec	—	—	—
Main (keep intensity between 60%-80% 1RM and velocity loss at 20%-30%)		EXERCISE	SETS	REPS, TIME	REST	TEMPO	VBT VELOCITY (M/SEC)
	1a	Incline T-row	5	3 reps	—	Explosive	0.40-0.50
	1b	Quadruped walkout	3	5 reps	—	—	—
	1c	Side-lying external rotation	3	10 reps each side	1 min	—	—
	2a	Push-up	5	5 reps	—	Explosive	0.40-0.50
	2b	Half-kneeling cable lift	3	8 reps per side	—	—	—
	2c	Split stance ER hold	2	5 reps per side	1 min	—	—
	3a	Suspension row	4	5 reps	—	Explosive	0.40-0.50
	3b	Hip-flow circuit	2	1 min	1 min	—	—

SAMPLE MAXIMAL STRENGTH (ABSOLUTE STRENGTH) LOWER-BODY PROGRAM FOR DAYS 1 AND 3

Warm-up		EXERCISE	SETS	TIME	REST	TEMPO	VBT VELOCITY (M/SEC)
	1	Airdyne bike	1	5 min	—	—	—

Power plyometrics		EXERCISE	SETS	REPS, TIME	REST	TEMPO	VBT VELOCITY (M/SEC)
	1a	Weighted vest countermovement jump	3	5 reps per side	—	Explosive	—
	1b	Rotary 6-cone drill	2	30 sec	1 min	—	—
	2a	Lateral power step-up	3	5 reps per side	—	Explosive	—
	2b	Shoulder tap	2	10 reps per side	1 min	—	—

Main (keep intensity between 80%-95% 1RM and velocity loss at 20%-30%)		EXERCISE	SETS	REPS, TIME	REST	TEMPO	VBT VELOCITY (M/SEC)
	1a	Trap bar deadlift	5	3 reps	—	2-0-0	0.30-0.50
	1b	Core stability at release	3	8 reps	—	—	—
	1c	Wall dribble	3	4 reps	3 min	—	—
	2a	Reverse lunge (dumbbell or barbell)	5	3 reps per side	—	2-0-0	0.30-0.50
	2b	Wide-stance cable rotation	3	8 reps per side	—	—	—
	2c	Prone internal rotation	3	8 reps	3 min	—	—
	3a	Single leg deadlift	4	3 reps per side	—	2-0-0	0.30-0.50
	3b	Shoulder tube	2	30 sec	3 min	—	—

SAMPLE MAXIMAL STRENGTH (ABSOLUTE STRENGTH) UPPER-BODY PROGRAM FOR DAYS 2 AND 4

Warm-up		EXERCISE	SETS	TIME	REST	TEMPO	VBT VELOCITY (M/SEC)
	1	Tempo run	8	30 sec	30 sec	—	—
Power plyometrics		**EXERCISE**	**SETS**	**REPS, TIME**	**REST**	**TEMPO**	**VBT VELOCITY (M/SEC)**
	1a	Split stance recoil slam	3	6 reps	—	Explosive	—
	1b	Suspension deep-squat breathing	2	10-15 sec	—	—	—
	2a	Medicine ball step-back shovel pass	3	5 reps per side	—	Explosive	—
	2b	One-arm doorway pectoral minor stretch	3	30 sec	—	—	—
Main (keep intensity between 80%-95% 1RM and velocity loss at 20%-30%)		**EXERCISE**	**SETS**	**REPS, DISTANCE, TIME**	**REST**	**TEMPO**	**VBT VELOCITY (M/SEC)**
	1a	One-arm dumbbell row	5	3 reps per side	—	2-0-0	0.30-0.40
	1b	Quadruped walkout	3	5 reps	—	—	—
	1c	Split stance external rotation hold	3	5 reps	3 min	—	—
	2a	Eccentric barbell bench press	5	3 reps	—	2-0-0	0.30-0.40
	2b	Waiter's walk	3	20 yd (18 m) per direction	—	—	—
	2c	Prone hip rotator stretch	2	30 sec	3 min	—	—
	3a	Incline T-row	4	3 reps	—	2-0-0	0.30-0.40
	3b	Band lateral stretch	3	30 sec	3 min	—	—
Conditioning		**EXERCISE**	**SETS**	**TIME**	**REST**	**TEMPO**	**VBT VELOCITY (M/SEC)**
	1	Sled sprint	5	6 sec	1 min	Explosive	—

The bottom line is that by creating gains in submaximal and maximal strengths in phase III, we can improve inter- and intramuscular coordination, respectively. Refining these neural outputs through increasing strength in phase III ultimately becomes gains in power, power endurance, and muscular endurance in phase IV. To create quick, explosive athletes requires working within the correct VBT strength zones, which creates the essential adaptations for developing higher activation of the type II fast-twitch fibers.

Late Off-Season and Preseason: Transfer to Sport-Specific Power

This chapter centers on phase IV, during which the different types of strength that have built up in previous phases of the off-season begin to transfer into the athlete's specific sport. Training sport-specific power involves learning to apply strength at faster rates (power) and for a specific period of time (power endurance) in preparation for competition. It also includes knowing the different types of sport-specific power and their correlating velocities and velocity losses.

This chapter also discusses training the different types of muscular endurance for athletes getting ready to compete in field sports and longer events, such as track and field and marathons. Because much of phase IV addresses power and power endurance (capacity), monitoring percentages of loss of both bar and body speeds as well as power output with VBT becomes more than ever a focal point in the weight room. Olympic lifting and the advantages and disadvantages of using mean, propulsive, and peak velocities when training these more ballistic movements are also discussed.

MAIN GOALS FOR LATE OFF-SEASON AND PRESEASON TRAINING

The following are the main goals when transferring off-season gains to sport.

Transfer Strength Gains Into Sport-Specific Power and Muscular Endurance

Depending on the sport, the maximal strength phase of training should be followed by one of these three fundamental options for conversion to sport:

- *Alactic power.* This type of power depends on the ATP-PC (creatine phosphate) system and provides energy for high-intensity movements that last between 1 and 10 seconds. This is the main type of power necessary for baseball, football, and the throwing and short sprinting events in track and field.
- *Lactic power.* This type of power relies on the lactic acid (anaerobic glycolysis) system and provides energy for high-intensity movements lasting between approximately 8 and 20 seconds. This is the main type of power needed in most field sports, short swimming events, and sprinting events in track and field.
- *Power endurance.* We not only have to train explosively to train power in sport but also have to be able to do it over and over again during actual competition. When training for power endurance, we are calling on all three energy systems—the ATP-PC, lactic acid, and aerobic systems—all working together to get the exercise done.

Improve Heart Efficiency and Lactate Threshold

Endurance sports are generally performed at submaximal paces in order to tolerate longer durations, and, therefore, the tension in the muscles is lower. The CNS first recruits both the slow- and fast-twitch muscle fibers that are adapted to function over longer durations. This, in turn, increases both the size of the heart's left ventricle and the heart's stroke volume. This process also enables the body to make better use of fat as fuel, thus sparing the storing and disposal of glycogen, and it conditions the body to reuse lactic acid more efficiently. Upon completion of the strength phase, we need to train muscular endurance in conjunction with power for sports that require strength to be expressed for longer periods of time (e.g., track and field and swimming events lasting over

30 seconds). This type of power relies primarily on the aerobic system and provides energy for moderate-to-high–intensity movements lasting longer than two minutes (e.g., field sports, swimming at distances greater than 100 yards [91 m], longer running events, and triathlons).

Monitor Velocity Loss to Train Explosive Power and Power Endurance

While the usage of accelerometers and LPTs to monitor velocity loss plays a key role in most aspects of training, it is most crucial in phase IV for training different types of power and power endurance (see figure 10.1). If velocity or power losses exceed 10 to 15 percent of the first rep of the set, this tells us a few things:

- The athlete is not truly being powerful on every rep—most likely due to fatigue.
- Rest intervals may need to be attenuated (made longer).
- Power endurance is not truly being trained, and the set has basically turned into a really difficult conditioning session.

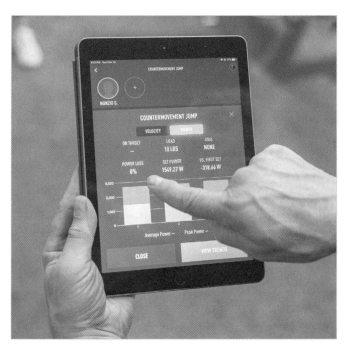

Figure 10. 1 Accelerometers and LPTs play a key role in most aspects of training for monitoring velocity loss and are especially important in phase IV for training different types of power and power endurance.

Alactic and lactic power and power endurance should never be trained in a fatigued state. If an athlete is not well rested between sets, recruitment patterns will diminish, causing the athlete to learn slower, less efficient movement patterns. For this reason, when training power, velocity or power losses of less than 10 percent (under 15 percent for power endurance) are used for ensuring good quality reps and higher recruitment patterns. This leads to better gains in speed and, ultimately, the continued production of power in both strength-speed and speed-strength ranges.

Table 10.1 provides a list of specific types of power that are trained in phase IV and the previously discussed primary energy systems that are based on the different durations and intensities of work being done.

Table 10.1 SPECIFIC POWER NEEDS BASED ON WORK OR DURATION OF EVENT

DURATION OF WORK OR EVENT	SAMPLE EVENT	WORK INTENSITY	MAIN ENERGY SYSTEMS USED	SPECIFIC POWER TRAINED
<10 sec	Shot put or baseball	Maximum to explosive	ATP-PC system	Alactic power
10 sec-1 min	Butterfly swim: 50 yd (46 m)	Maximum	Lactic acid system	Lactic power, power endurance
1-2 min	Track: 800 m	High	Lactic acid and aerobic systems	Power endurance, muscular endurance (short)
2-8 min	Track: 5,000 m	Moderate to high	Aerobic system	Muscular endurance (long)

PROGRAMMING FOR SPORT-SPECIFIC ADAPTATIONS

This section includes programming for the four training adaptations used when beginning to transfer strength to sport: alactic power, lactic power, power endurance, and muscular endurance (short and long). Remember, the difference between training power and power endurance from a programming standpoint is in the duration of the work–rest ratios used. Therefore, different sports require different amounts of training time for each trait.

Here is a brief recap. Whether it is a soccer player running and kicking, a swimmer jumping off the block, or an MMA athlete in the ring, all sports (with the possible exception of a marathon runner) require power. Each sport uses a different type of power that needs to be produced for different amounts of time. When training alactic power, lactic power, or power endurance, peak power is produced in either the strength-speed or speed-strength zones. As described in chapter 4, these two zones blend into one another as different athletes produce their highest power numbers in either of these two zones. For this reason, VBT is also used for monitoring power output and loss. This helps tell us not only where athletes are producing their highest power numbers but also if they are maintaining power from set to set.

Ballistic movements such as the Olympic lifts may also be introduced in phase IV. Remember, once faster movements become necessary, the use of ballistic movements becomes paramount. These are exercises where the implement (bar, ball, or body) is thrown into the air. The exercises lack a deceleration component, so using *mean* velocity may not be the best choice for tracking velocities because mean velocity measures the entire concentric movement. When tracking ballistic movements such as hang cleans and snatches, force is only imparted on the bar up to the second pull. The fact that the athlete is never locking out or grinding out a rep (decelerating) when the movement is done properly makes calculating with mean velocity a bit pointless. For this reason, I choose

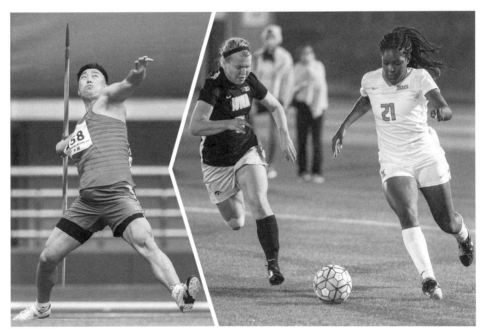

Dependent upon the sport, different types of power need to be produced for different amounts of time and train either the alactic or lactic system.

(a) Xinhua/Jia Yuchen via Getty Images; (b) © Human Kinetics

to use peak velocity (PV) because it only measures the quickest 10 milliseconds of the movement, taking the deceleration component out of the measurement completely.

If I had my ultimate choice and everyone had a Tendo unit, I would use mean propulsive velocity (MPV). Unfortunately, few units on the market have this feature available, so PV is what most of them use to measure Olympic lifts. The more time we can spend developing force, the higher velocities we can expect. For this reason, taller athletes with longer lever arms should expect higher velocities during Olympic lifts and other ballistic movements most of the time. See the table on page 55 of chapter 4 for differences in velocity according to height of two sample Olympic lifts—the snatch and the hang clean.

Phase IV: Alactic and Lactic Power (Weeks 1 Through 4)

The two main differences between alactic and lactic power are the amount of time power is being produced and the energy systems being trained, and they have less to do with velocities that are prescribed. Even though the duration of power expression is longer, *the same velocity can be used when training lactic power as when training alactic power and vice versa. This is dependent upon the athlete's level of maximal strength and power endurance.* For this reason, as mentioned earlier, I like to monitor power output and velocity loss with the VBT device instead of, or along with, velocity to utilize a load where the athlete is producing their greatest "power output" while maintaining velocity losses <10% within the set.

That being said, let's take a closer look at these two types of power.

Alactic Power

TRAINING PARAMETERS

Intensity	40%-80% 1RM (wherever peak power is achieved)
VBT velocity	0.50-1.0 m/sec (accelerative strength/strength-speed)
VBT velocity or power loss	<10%
Tempo	Explosive
Reps	2-5 (<10 sec)
Sets	3-8
Rest	2-3 min
Frequency of training	2-3 times per week for full body; 3-4 times per week for upper- and lower-splits

PROGRAMMING

SAMPLE ALACTIC POWER FULL-BODY PROGRAM

Warm-up		EXERCISE	SETS	TIME	REST	TEMPO	VBT VELOCITY (M/SEC)
	1	Tempo run	8	30 sec	1 min	—	—

Main (keep intensity between 40%-80% 1RM and velocity or power loss at <10%)		EXERCISE	SETS	REPS	REST	TEMPO	VBT VELOCITY (M/SEC)
	1	Trap bar deadlift	6	5	2 min	Explosive	Lower body: 0.75-1.0 Upper body: 0.60-0.80
	2	Half-kneeling reverse cable row	6	5	2 min	Explosive	Upper body: 0.60-0.80
	3	Split squat	6	5 per side	2 min	Explosive	Lower body: 0.75-1.0
	4	Dumbbell bench-floor press	6	5	2 min	Explosive	Upper body: 0.60-0.80

Core		EXERCISE	SETS	REPS	REST	TEMPO	VBT VELOCITY (M/SEC)
	1a	Dead bug	2	8 per side	—	—	—
	1b	Half-kneeling cable chop	2	6 per side	—	—	—
	1c	Shoulder tap	2	10 per side	1 min	—	—
Conditioning		EXERCISE	SETS	DISTANCE	REST	TEMPO	VBT VELOCITY (M/SEC)
	1	Buildup	5	30 yd (27 m)	2 min	—	—

Lactic Power

TRAINING PARAMETERS

Intensity	20-60% 1RM (wherever peak power is achieved)
VBT velocity	Lower body: 0.75-1.3 m/sec Upper body: 0.60-1.0 m/sec (strength-speed and speed-strength)
VBT velocity or power loss	<10%
Tempo	Explosive
Reps	12-30
Sets	3-8
Rest	4-12 min
Frequency of training	2-3 times per week for full body; 3-4 times per week for upper- and lower-splits

PROGRAMMING

SAMPLE LACTIC POWER FULL-BODY PROGRAM

Warm-up		EXERCISE	SETS	TIME	REST	TEMPO	VBT VELOCITY (M/SEC)
	1	Tempo run	8	30 sec	—	—	—
Main (keep intensity between 20%-60% 1RM and velocity or power loss at <10%)		**EXERCISE**	**SETS**	**REPS**	**REST**	**TEMPO**	**VBT VELOCITY (M/SEC)**
	1	Trap bar deadlift	3	12	4 min	Explosive	Lower body: 0.75-1.0
	2	Prone seal row	3	15	3 min	Explosive	Upper body: 0.60-0.80
	3	Front squat	3	12	4 min	Explosive	Lower body: 0.75-1.0
	4	Dumbbell bench-floor press	3	15	3 min	Explosive	Upper body: 0.60-0.80
Core		**EXERCISE**	**SETS**	**REPS**	**REST**	**TEMPO**	**VBT VELOCITY (M/SEC)**
	1a	Dead bug	2	8 per side	—	—	—
	1b	Half-kneeling cable chop	2	6 per side	—	—	—
	1c	Shoulder tap	2	10 per side	1 min	—	—
Conditioning		**EXERCISE**	**SETS**	**DISTANCE**	**REST**	**TEMPO**	**VBT VELOCITY (M/SEC)**
	1	Buildup	5	30 yd (27 m)	2 min	—	—

Phase IV: Power Endurance (Weeks 5 Through 8)

In some sports, especially the field sports, athletes must apply a high degree of power repetitively after only a few moments of game interruption (Bompa and Buzzichelli 2015). This is otherwise known as power endurance (capacity). The duration athletes need to produce these expressions of power depends on the sport. Note: Athletes who already possess a high degree of power may begin training power endurance in weeks 1 through 5. However, most athletes—especially novice athletes—must first work on power expression during weeks 1 through 4 of this phase before moving on to power endurance in weeks 5 through 8.

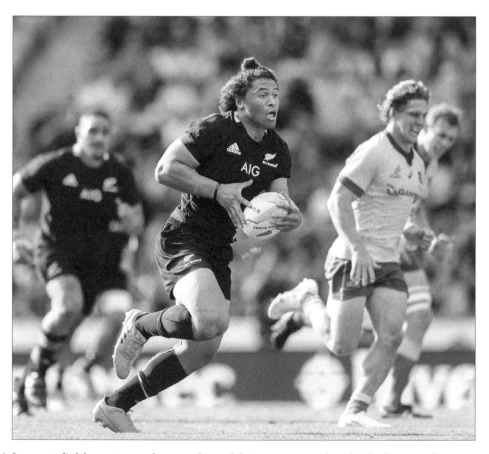

In most field sports, such as rugby, athletes must apply a high degree of power repetitively after only a few moments of game interruption, making power endurance a main focus in phase IV.

Anthony Au-Yeung/Getty Images

When training power endurance with sports such as baseball, throwing sports, and most field sports that require power to be produced with an average duration under 10 seconds (alactic power), we use a low number of reps (three to six). With sports such as wrestling and some field sports that require power to be produced with an average duration of 8 to 20 seconds (lactic power), we use a higher number of reps (12 to 30). These reps are performed and grouped into sets with short breaks of 5 to 20 seconds that coincide with the pace of their specific sport. We then group these sets into series or clusters of sets based on the volume, duration, and rest time required of the sport. The rest between series is somewhat long to allow for full recovery before beginning another series of sets. For example, an athlete performing four sets of five weighted jumps for two series would be written like this:

$$2 \times 4 \times 5$$

Similar to training for power, training for power endurance is also a time when more ballistic movements, such as Olympic lifts and jumps, as well as exercises that closely mimic the sport, can be used. PVs with VBT can also be used if so desired. See chapters 4 and 10 for more information on the use of ballistic movements and PV.

TRAINING PARAMETERS

Intensity*	20%-60% 1RM
VBT velocity**	0.75-1.0 m/sec (strength-speed) 1.0-1.3 m/sec (speed-strength)
VBT velocity or power loss	<10%
Tempo	Explosive
Series	2-4
Sets	3-6
Reps	Alactic power: 2-5 Lactic power: 12-30
Rest	5-20 sec between sets; 3-5 min between series (based on requirements of the sport)
Frequency of training	2-3 times per week for full body; 3-4 times per week for upper- and lower-splits

*This range is determined by the length of the set as well as the load at which athletes produce their peak power.

**Velocity used is dependent upon the strength and explosiveness of the athletes. Each athlete creates optimal power in a different part of the power zones (strength-speed and speed-strength).

PROGRAMMING

SAMPLE POWER ENDURANCE FULL-BODY PROGRAM

Warm-up		EXERCISE	SETS	TIME	REST	TEMPO	VBT VELOCITY (M/SEC)
	1	Jump rope	1	5 min	—	—	—

Main (keep intensity between 20%-60% 1RM and velocity or power loss <10%-15%)		EXERCISE	SERIES	SETS × REPS	REST	TEMPO	VBT VELOCITY (M/SEC)
	1	Power clean	3	3 × 5	4 min between series; 20 sec between sets	Explosive	1.5-2.0 m/sec (PV used on Olympic lifts)
	2	Trap bar jump (20%-40% of maximal strength)	2	5 × 5	4 min between series; 20 sec between sets	Explosive	1.0-1.3
	3	Kettlebell swing	2	5 × 5	4 min between series; 20 sec between sets	Explosive	1.0-1.3
	4	Barbell bench throw	2	5 × 5	4 min between series; 20 sec between series	Explosive	0.85-1.0

Core		EXERCISE	SETS	REPS, BREATH	REST	TEMPO	VBT VELOCITY (M/SEC)
	1a	Pallof press	2	8 reps per side	—	—	—
	1b	Wide-stance cable rotation	2	8 reps per side	—	—	—
	1c	Money maker	2	5 breaths	1 min	—	—

Conditioning		EXERCISE	SETS	TIME	REST	TEMPO	VBT VELOCITY (M/SEC)
	1	Sled sprint	5	8-10 sec	2 min	—	—

Phase IV: Muscular Endurance

Most sports involve an endurance component, and muscular endurance methods train both the neural and metabolic aspects specific to a sport (Parejo-Blanco et al. 2016). Muscular endurance—the ability to maintain both the work levels over extended periods of time and the sport's energy system requirements—is categorized into these three methods:

- *Short (lactic capacity).* The average duration is 30 seconds to 2 minutes, such as in the 100-yard butterfly (91 m).
- *Long (aerobic power).* The average duration is 2 to 8 minutes, such as in the 200-yard butterfly (183 m).
- *Extended (aerobic capacity).* The average duration is 8 to 10 minutes, such as in a marathon or triathlon.

Using set-rep schemes combined with VBT intensities allows the athlete to apply less force for a longer period of time when training muscular endurance. Note: Muscular endurance is not as much of a concern or priority with explosive sports that rely on alactic power (baseball or shot put) in which power expression is less than 10 seconds. For these sports, strength and power are the dominant traits being trained.

TRAINING PARAMETERS

SHORT (LACTIC CAPACITY)	Intensity	40%-60% 1RM
	VBT velocity*	Lower body: 0.75-1.0 m/sec Upper body: 0.60-.070 m/sec
	VBT velocity loss**	—
	Series	2-4
	Sets	2-6 (each exercise is a set)
	Time	30 sec-2 min
	Rest	5-20 sec between sets; 3-5 min between series
LONG (AEROBIC POWER)	Intensity	20%-40% 1RM
	VBT velocity*	Lower body: 1.0-1.3 m/sec Upper body: 0.85-1.0 m/sec
	VBT velocity loss**	—
	Series	2-4
	Sets	1-3 (each exercise is a set)
	Time	2-8 min
	Rest	2-3 min between sets; 2-4 min between series

Extended (aerobic capacity)***	Intensity	Body weight-30% 1RM (both lower- and upper-body)
	VBT velocity*	>1.3 m/sec
	VBT velocity loss**	—
	Series	1-3
	Sets	4-6 (each exercise is a set)
	Time	8-10 min
	Rest	1 min between sets; 2-3 min between series

*VBT intensities are used only as starting intensities in order to program correct loads.

**I do not program velocity losses when training muscular endurance because of working to capacity.

***I have included parameters for extended (aerobic capacity) to accommodate marathon and triathlon training. I have not included a training program because I feel it is beyond my expertise.

PROGRAMMING

SAMPLE MUSCULAR ENDURANCE SHORT FULL-BODY PROGRAM

Warm-up		EXERCISE	SETS	TIME	REST	TEMPO	VBT VELOCITY (M/SEC)
	1	Jump rope	3	2 min	1 min	—	—

Power plyometrics		EXERCISE	SETS	REPS	REST	TEMPO	VBT VELOCITY (M/SEC)
	1a	Sit-up to medicine ball overhead throw	2	5 per side	—	Explosive	—
	1b	Box jump	2	5 per side	1 min	Explosive	—
	2a	Sit-up to medicine ball chest pass	2	5 per side	—	Explosive	—
	2b	Power step-up	2	5 per side	1 min	Explosive	—

Phase IV: Muscular Endurance

Main (keep intensity between 40%-60% 1RM)		EXERCISE	SERIES	SETS × REPS OR TIME	REST	TEMPO	VBT VELOCITY (M/SEC)
	1	Split squat	2	4 × 30 sec	4 min between series; 15 sec between sets	Explosive	Lower body: 0.75-1.0
	2	Cable retraction to low row	2	4 × 30 sec	4 min between series; 15 sec between sets	—	Upper body: 0.60-0.70
	3	Band-resisted bench press	2	4 × 30 sec	4 min between series; 15 sec between sets	Explosive	Upper body: 0.60-0.70
	4	Triceps rope pull-down	2	4 × 30 sec	4 min between series; 15 sec between sets	Explosive	—
	5a	Half-kneeling cable lift	2	2 × 8 reps per side	30 sec	—	—
	5b	Side bridge	2	2 × 8 reps per side	1 min	—	—

SAMPLE MUSCULAR ENDURANCE LONG FULL-BODY PROGRAM

Warm-up		EXERCISE	SETS	TIME	REST	TEMPO	VBT (M/SEC)
	1	Jump rope	3	2 min	1 min	—	—
Power plyometrics		EXERCISE	SETS	REPS	REST	TEMPO	VBT VELOCITY (M/SEC)
	1a	Sit-up to medicine ball overhead throw	2	5 per side	—	Explosive	—
	1b	Box jump	2	5 per side	1 min	Explosive	—
	2a	Sit-up to medicine ball chest pass	2	5 per side	—	Explosive	—
	2b	Power step-up	2	5 per side	1 min	Explosive	—

Main (keep intensity between 20%-40% 1RM)		EXERCISE	SERIES	SETS × TIME	REST	TEMPO	VBT VELOCITY (M/SEC)
	1	Bench hip bridge	2	2 × 1 min	4 min between series; 10 sec between sets	Explosive	Lower body: 1.0-1.3
	2	Lat pull-down	2	2 × 1 min	4 min between series; 10 sec between sets	Explosive	Upper body: 0.85-1.0
	3	Back squat	2	2 × 1 min	4 min between series; 10 sec between sets	Explosive	Upper body: 0.85-1.0
	4	Band-resisted bench press	2	2 × 1 min	4 min between series; 10 sec between sets	Explosive	Upper body: 0.85-1.0
	5	Seated dumbbell biceps curl	2	2 × 1 min	4 min between series; 10 sec between sets	Explosive	—

When transitioning off-season strength gains to more sport-specific movements, training traits such as power and muscular endurance is vital to successfully entering the competitive period. The focal point (alactic or lactic power, power endurance, or muscular endurance) in this phase is determined by the sport. Many field sports, such as lacrosse and soccer, require time spent in all three traits, whereas more explosive sports, such as baseball or throwing events in track and field, lean heavily on the side of power. No matter what trait is being trained, small volumes of maximal strength should be included and maintained because maximal strength is the foundation for all other types of strength.

In-Season: Strength and Power Maintenance

This chapter looks at some of the different circumstances that need to be considered as well as the different methods of training for them when building an in-season program in phase V. I often tell athletes that programming during the season is like trying to hit a moving target. This is primarily due to the fact that competition has started, and schedules can be a bit sporadic. As a result, staying consistent within a weekly training program becomes almost impossible. In this chapter, some of the hurdles coaches face when programming for athletes in-season are addressed:

- The management of training residuals
- The calculation of strength proportions required for the sport
- The use of undulating (nonlinear) periodization

In most sports, the only type of strength training performed in-season is sport-specific power training. As a result, maximum strength, power endurance (capacity), and muscular endurance are often overlooked. This is usually accompanied by a steady decline in training adaptations beginning somewhere after the first three to six weeks of play. For this reason, both athletes and coaches need to incorporate various degrees of submaximal and maximal strengths, power, power endurance, and muscular endurance, when applicable, into their program during the competitive phase. How much of each adaptation is prescribed in an athlete's in-season program is based mostly on what that athlete's particular sport requires (covered later in this chapter regarding proportions of strength).

MAIN GOALS FOR IN-SEASON MAINTENANCE

I always tell my athletes that once the season begins, and the majority of time is spent playing our specific sport, what we are really doing is managing a controlled fall. In other words, playing sports *technically* makes athletes better at playing their sport, but it does not make them stronger or even able to maintain specific training adaptations as the season progresses.

In order to keep up with the demands of the competitive period, a few things must be addressed in terms of programming. Let's take a look at what I believe are the main goals for creating a good in-season training program.

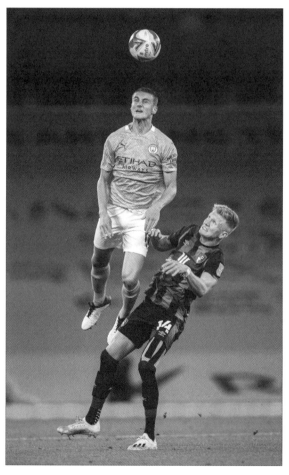

Maintaining strength during the in-season is like managing a controlled fall.

Visionhaus/Getty Images

Management of Training Residuals

To create a successful in-season program, the first important step is to understand that what playing the sport helps to develop and sustain differs from what the athlete still needs in order to be successful in that sport (Winkelman 2012). Training residual represents the length of time a specific adaptation stays with the athlete once the training stimulus is removed (Winkelman 2012). For example, back squatting to stay strong is not a trained quality while playing a field sport, but it greatly increases the athlete's ability to perform in that sport. Thus, this must be a focus of any effective in-season training program in order to maintain strength and keep play at a high level throughout the entire season. Table. 11.1 shows the training residual time frame of specific adaptations (Issurin 2008), or, in other words, how long a particular adaptation stays with the athlete once game play begins.

Table 11.1 TRAINING RESIDUAL TIME FRAME FOR SPECIFIC ADAPTATIONS

ADAPTIVE QUALITY	TRAINING RESIDUAL TIME FRAME
Muscular endurance and aerobic strength	30 days (+/– 5 days)
Maximal strength	30 days (+/– 5 days)
Power	18 days (+/– 5 days)
Power endurance	15 days (+/– 5 days)
Speed	5 days (+/– 3 days)

Note that the first two adaptive qualities—muscular endurance and aerobic and maximal strength—last longer once training stops. These are the two traits that rely on anatomical adaptations such as mitochondrial density (tissue prep, hypertrophy) for the aerobic system and myofibril density (hypertrophy and lean muscle mass) for maximal strength (Issurin 2008). The fact that these adaptations need to degrade before we see a decrease in that particular system allows them to last longer once training them stops. As a result, they do not need to be trained as frequently as traits such as power, power endurance, and speed. (Note: I have not included training "speed" in this text because I do not include it in my programming—it is the one trait that is constantly being trained in-season through game play and practices and does not rely on the use of VBT.)

In addition to cessation of training quality, other limiting factors that can cause specific traits to decline more quickly include the following:

- *Inefficient amount of time spent in the preparatory period.* The shorter the time you spend on a particular quality, the less time it stays with you. The preparatory period is when tissue prep, hypertrophy, and submaximal and maximal strengths are the main focus of development. For example, an athlete who starts the off-season training two months late and is only able to spend six weeks in the preparatory period will more than likely see strength qualities decline more quickly once constant game play starts than an athlete who spends 8 to 12 weeks in this period. Consequently, the anatomical adaptations built in the preparatory period are not developed to as high a degree, causing adaptations to decline at a faster rate in-season (Issurin 2008). For this reason, I use linear or block periodization as opposed to undulating periodization in the early off-season in order to allow more time to be spent in each phase (see chapter 7).

- *Applying undulating (nonlinear) periodization too early in the off-season.* This goes hand in hand with the first factor listed, and it greatly reduces the saturation period, or the amount of time working on a specific quality.

Calculate Specific Strength Proportions Required for the Sport

Athletes in most sports need to maintain maximum strength, power, and power endurance. Because competition and practices during the in-season limit the time devoted to training, these adaptations must all be trained together week to week, day to day, or sometimes even within the same day. All traits are important to optimize performance, and for this reason, *one should not take priority over the other.* For example, throwers in track and field and linemen in American football must maintain maximum strength during the competitive phase with a roughly equal proportion between maximum strength and power. Most athletes in endurance sports should maintain different percentages of maximum strength, power endurance, and muscular endurance depending on the sport or position they play.

Table 11.2 provides the in-season ratios (percentages) of total volume (load, sets, rest) for different adaptations used in different sports. These ratios are based on Tudor Bompa's *Periodization Training for Sports* (Bompa and Buzzichelli 2015), although I have changed some of the

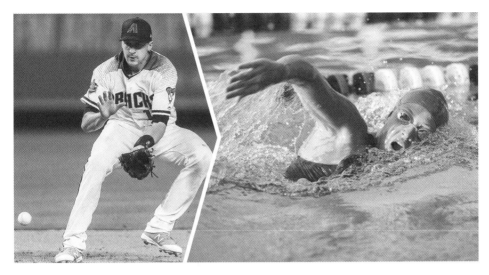

Different traits dominate different sports. For example, *(a)* a shortstop requires predominantly power, while *(b)* a 200-meter freestyle swimmer is predominantly power endurance—and muscular endurance—based.

(a) Adam Bow/Icon Sportswire via Getty Images; *(b)* © EyeWire/Getty Images

Table 11.2 EXAMPLE PROPORTIONS OF IN-SEASON STRENGTH BASED ON THE NEEDS OF THE SPORT

SPORT OR EVENT	MAXIMUM STRENGTH	POWER (ALACTIC AND LACTIC POWER)	POWER ENDURANCE	MUSCULAR ENDURANCE
Baseball (pitcher)	40%	40%	20%	—
Baseball (position)	30%	60%	10%	—
Swimming (100 m)	40%	40%	20%	—
Swimming (200 m)	10%	10%	30%	50%
Soccer or lacrosse	30%	40%	20%	10%
MMA	10%	40%	30%	20%

Adapted from T.O. Bompa and C.A. Buzzichelli, *Periodization Training for Sports*, 3rd ed. (Champaign, IL: Human Kinetics, 2015), 312.

metrics slightly based on my experience training these particular types of athletes. In this text, Bompa includes a list of all sports, whereas I have listed only a few as examples, and I have changed the percentages a bit according to my own personal experiences with the athletes and for the sports that I train. I have used this information when creating my in-season protocol for years with great success. I suggest you refer to *Periodization Training for Sports* if you desire to acquire ratios for the athletes and sports that pertain to you.

IN-SEASON PROGRAMMING FOR SPORT

As we learned in chapter 7, undulating (nonlinear) periodization is a type of programming with a dynamic scheme that allows for weekly or daily fluctuations in training parameters and methods while still having a base structure to build from. This type of periodization is used to build a strong foundation of multiple strength adaptations at the same time. It is also used during the season when practices and games begin to take time away from in-gym training. With undulating periodization, multiple training adaptations are used in order to train in the fewest training sessions possible. As a result, when training different adaptations in the same session, both velocity losses and power losses can be

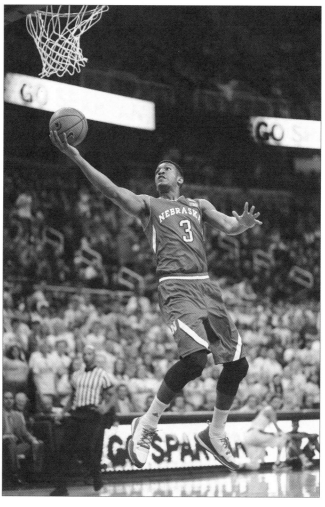

Sports such as basketball require as much as three times the power to be maintained in-season as compared to maximum strength.

Rey Del Rio/Getty Images

monitored at the same time using VBT. This is also, in my opinion, what makes undulating periodization a more efficient type of programming and is the type of periodization I use in table 11.3 of a sample microcycle program for a basketball player (an athlete in a power sport). Note: While each day focuses on a different trait, we will not get into the amount of volume in each day. Chapter 12 includes this as well as sample programs.

TABLE 11.3 SAMPLE TWO-DAY IN-SEASON FULL-BODY PROGRAM FOR A HIGH SCHOOL OR COLLEGIATE BASKETBALL PLAYER (MAXIMUM STRENGTH: 20 PERCENT; POWER: 60 PERCENT; POWER ENDURANCE: 20 PERCENT)

DAY 1: MAXIMUM STRENGTH AND POWER						
Note that I am monitoring both velocity and power losses in day 1 according to the type of exercise being performed. This is because we are incorporating undulating periodization, so we are training multiple traits in one session. We are monitoring velocity losses of 20 to 30 percent when training strength exercises, but we are looking at power losses of less than 10 percent in order to maintain power output when performing explosive exercises.						
Warm-up		EXERCISE	SETS	TIME	REST	TEMPO	VBT VELOCITY (M/SEC)
	1	Tempo run	8	30 sec	—	Explosive	—
Main (keep intensity at 80%-90% 1RM and 20%-30% velocity loss for strength exercises, and 40%-60% 1RM with <10% power loss when performing power exercises)		EXERCISE	SETS	REPS	REST	TEMPO	VBT VELOCITY (M/SEC)
	1	Strength: back squat	3	3	3 min, or as needed	2-0-0	0.40-0.50
	2	Strength: barbell bench press	3	3	3 min, or as needed	2-0-0	0.35-0.45
	3	Power: trap bar deadlift	4	4	2 min	Explosive	0.75-1.0
	4	Power: bilateral cable row	4	4	2 min	Explosive	0.60-0.70
	5	Power: lateral dumbbell lunge	4	4	2 min	Explosive	0.75-1.0
Core		EXERCISE	SETS	REPS	REST	TEMPO	VBT VELOCITY (M/SEC)
	1a	Dead bug	2	6 per side		—	—
	1b	Pallof press with hold	2	6 per side	1 min	0-5-0	—
DAY 2: POWER ENDURANCE AND POWER						
Warm-up		EXERCISE	SETS	REPS	REST	TEMPO	VBT VELOCITY (M/SEC)
	1	Mobility circuit	1	—	—	—	—

Main (keep intensity between 40%-60% 1RM for power, 20-40% 1RM for power endurance, and power losses at <10%)		EXERCISE	SERIES	SETS × REPS	REST	TEMPO	VBT VELOCITY (M/SEC)
	1	Power endurance: trap bar jump	2	6 × 3	30 sec between sets; 3 min between series	Explosive	1.8-2.0 (use peak velocities)
	2	Power endurance: barbell bench throw	2	6 × 3	30 sec between sets; 3 min between series	Explosive	1.8-2.0

		EXERCISE	SETS	REPS	REST	TEMPO	VBT VELOCITY (M/SEC)
	3	Power: back squat	4	4	30 sec	Explosive	0.75-1.0
	4	Power: band-assisted push-up	4	4	30 sec	Explosive	0.60-0.70
	5	Power: split squat	4	4	30 sec	Explosive	0.75-1.0

Core		EXERCISE	SETS	REPS	REST	TEMPO	VBT VELOCITY (M/SEC)
	1a	Dead bug	2	8 per side	—	—	—
	1b	Half-kneeling cable chop	2	6 per side	—	—	—

The benefits of strength to athletic performance are experienced as long as the neuromuscular system maintains the cellular adaptations induced by training (Bompa and Buzzichelli 2015). If strength training is ceased, the benefits soon decrease as the contractile properties of the muscles diminish and a noticeable decline in athletic performance begins to take effect. This is not usually a problem early on in the season while strength gains from off-season training are still lingering, but as the season continues, training residuals start to diminish stripping an athlete of strength, power, and endurance. Even slight declines in any or all of these traits will have a negative effect on the athlete's ability to perform at optimum levels.

To avoid detraining, athletes must implement sport-specific strength programs during the in-season (competitive phase). This (most times, due to time constraints) involves training different qualities within the same week and thus makes undulating periodization a more efficient choice.

CHAPTER

12

Sample Programming

This final chapter provides a few different examples of full-body programs and how I incorporate VBT into the various phases of an athlete's yearly plan. Even though these are examples of full-body programs, they can be divided into upper- and lower-splits to accrue more volume per body part.

The first three phases of programming in the preparatory period are designed for *all athletes*, regardless of sport. The programs are designed to prepare athletes for more sport-specific training in phases IV and V as the competitive season draws near. For example, a field athlete requires different amounts of every type of strength adaptation as opposed to a javelin thrower or baseball player who only needs to focus on maximal strength and power. For this reason, the sections on phases IV and V provide sample programming for various sports, while the sections on phases I, II, and III provide sample programming that applies to any type of athlete.

To recap, the VBT velocities in all of the sample programs are general ranges. Each athlete is different and will fall somewhere in those ranges. The ranges are based on an individual athlete's force–velocity profile, which should be performed prior to the initial training program (see chapter 5). If a profile is not possible, the ranges listed in the training parameters tables have worked well for me over the years, reaping beneficial results. The velocity ranges provided in phases I and II (tissue prep and hypertrophy) are used only as starting points to acquire an accurate starting load. With the amount of time spent under tension in these phases, velocity cannot be expected, nor is it desirable to maintain. In all phases, the velocities will vary somewhere within the provided ranges as a result of the athlete's force–velocity profile. Also, VBT should not be used on all exercises—only the core lifts will include velocities.

Similarly, the velocity-loss ranges serve as a guide to ensure that adequate amounts of stress are applied to muscle fibers to create the desired size and strength adaptations during the first three phases. In addition, we also use the prescribed power losses for training power and muscular endurance in phase IV and during the in-season to ensure that we are using adequate rest periods to maintain speed and power throughout the exercise. (See chapter 6 on velocity loss if you need to review further.)

I encourage readers to use the following sample programs as templates for creating your own programs. As you become more efficient with programming and comfortable reading VBT velocities and velocity losses, it will be easier for you to design programs that address the specific needs of your athletes in their respective sports.

Phase I: Early Off-Season

Tissue Prep

After a long season and a short recovery period, the preparatory period begins. This first phase tissue-prep does exactly what it states: It prepares the tissues and tendons for the upcoming heavier work in phases II and III.

GOALS

- Strengthening the tendons (tensile strength), especially in low positions
- Regrooving good movement patterns in the weight room

TRAINING PARAMETERS

Training intensity	40%-60% 1RM (increase weekly)
VBT velocity (concentric phase)	0.75-1.0 m/sec (starting velocity only)
VBT velocity loss	30%-40%
Tempo	3-1-0, 3-2-0, 4-2-0
Reps	12-15 down to 8 (decrease weekly by 2 reps, and incorporate velocity rep scheme)
Sets	2-4 per exercise
Rest	1-2 min between sets
Frequency of training	2-4 times per week

SAMPLE PROGRAM

SAMPLE TISSUE PREP FULL-BODY PROGRAM

Warm-up		EXERCISE	SETS	TIME	REST	TEMPO	VBT VELOCITY (M/SEC)
	1	Airdyne bike	1	10 min	—	—	—

Main (keep intensity between 40%-60% 1RM and velocity loss at 30%-40%)		EXERCISE	SETS	REPS, TIME	REST	TEMPO	VBT VELOCITY (M/SEC)
	1a	Single-leg deadlift	3	15 reps per side	—	3-2-0	0.75-1.0
	1b	Prone hip rotator stretch	2	30 sec per side	90 sec	—	—
	2a	Military press	3	15 reps	—	4-2-0	0.60-0.70
	2b	Side-lying cross-body stretch	2	30 sec per side	90 sec	—	—
	3a	Front squat	3	15 reps	—	4-2-0	0.75-1.0
	3b	Tri-planar hamstring stretch	2	30 sec per side	90 sec	—	—
	4a	Upright row	3	15 reps	—	4-2-0	0.60-0.70
	4b	Band lat stretch	2	30 sec per side	90 sec	—	—
	5a	Leg curl	3	15 reps	—	3-2-0	0.75-1.0
	5b	Figure 4 stretch	2	30 sec per side	90 sec	—	—

Core		EXERCISE	SETS	REPS, TIME	REST	TEMPO	VBT VELOCITY (M/SEC)
	1a	V sit-up	3	30 sec	—	—	—
	1b	Half-kneeling cable lift	3	12 reps per side	1 min	—	—

Phase II: Early Off-Season

Hypertrophy

Once tissue and tendon strength have been addressed, the focus turns to increasing muscle size and strength (lean body mass).

GOALS

- Increasing the size of the muscle cross-sectional area fibers of the type I low-threshold muscle fibers (hypertrophy I)
- Increasing the size of the muscle cross-sectional area fibers of the type II high-threshold muscle fibers (hypertrophy II)
- Increasing the storage capacity for high-energy substrates and enzymes (recovery)

TRAINING PARAMETERS

Training intensity	Hypertrophy I: 40%-60% 1RM (increase weekly)
	Hypertrophy II: 75%-85% 1RM (increase weekly)
VBT velocity	Hypertrophy I: 0.75-.1.0 m/sec (starting velocities only)
	Hypertrophy II: 0.40-0.60 m/sec (starting velocities only)
VBT velocity loss	Hypertrophy I: 40%-50%
	Hypertrophy II: 10%-20%
Tempo	Hypertrophy I: 3-0-0, 4-0-0
	Hypertrophy II: 1-0-0, 2-0-0
Reps	Hypertrophy I: 16 down to 10 (decrease weekly by 2 reps; incorporate velocity loss into rep scheme)
	Hypertrophy II: 10 down to 5 (decrease weekly by 2 reps; incorporate velocity loss into rep scheme)
Sets	Hypertrophy I: 3-5 per exercise
	Hypertrophy II: 3-8 per exercise
Rest	Hypertrophy I: 1-3 min
	Hypertrophy II: 2-5 min
Frequency of training	2-4 times per week

SAMPLE PROGRAMS

SAMPLE HYPERTROPHY I FULL-BODY PROGRAM

Warm-up		EXERCISE	SETS	TIME	REST	TEMPO	VBT VELOCITY (M/SEC)
	1	Spin bike or Airdyne bike	1	5 min	—	—	—

Power plyometrics		EXERCISE	SETS	REPS, TIME	REST	TEMPO	VBT VELOCITY (M/SEC)
	1a	Medicine ball slam: 8-10 lb (4-5 kg)	3	8 reps	—	Explosive	—
	1b	Band lat stretch	2	30 sec per side	1 min	—	—
	2a	Box jump	3	6 reps	—	Explosive	—
	2b	T-spine rotation	2	8 reps per side	1 min	—	—

Main (keep intensity between 40%-60% 1RM and 40%-50% velocity loss)		EXERCISE	SETS	REPS, TIME	REST	TEMPO	VBT VELOCITY (M/SEC)
	1a	Straight bar deadlift	4	12 reps	—	3-0-0	0.75-0.80
	1b	Band hamstring stretch	3	30 sec	2 min	—	—
	2a	One-arm dumbbell row	4	12 reps per side	—	4-0-0	0.75-0.80
	2b	Cat-camel stretch	3	10 reps	2 min	—	—
	3a	Barbell front squat	4	12 reps	—	3-0-0	0.75-0.80
	3b	Sumo stretch	3	30 sec	2 min	—	—
	4a	Loaded push-up	4	14 reps	—	4-0-0	0.75-0.80
	4b	Doorway pec stretch	3	30 sec	2 min	—	—

Core		EXERCISE	SETS	REPS, TIME	REST	TEMPO	VBT VELOCITY (M/SEC)
	1a	Plank	3	30 sec	—	—	—
	1b	Side plank	3	8 reps per side	1 min	—	—

SAMPLE HYPERTROPHY II FULL-BODY PROGRAM

Warm-up		EXERCISE	SETS	TIME	REST	TEMPO	VBT VELOCITY (M/SEC)
	1	Spin bike or Airdyne bike	1	5 min	—	—	—

Power plyometrics		EXERCISE	SETS	REPS, TIME	REST	TEMPO	VBT VELOCITY (M/SEC)
	1a	Medicine ball slam: 8-10 lb (4-5 kg)	3	8 reps	—	Explosive	—
	1b	Band lat stretch	2	30 sec per side	1 min	—	—
	2a	Box jump	3	6 reps	—	Explosive	—
	2b	T-spine rotation	2	8 reps per side	1 min	—	—

Main (keep intensity between 75%-85% 1RM and velocity loss at 10%-20%)		EXERCISE	SETS	REPS, TIME	REST	TEMPO	VBT VELOCITY (M/SEC)
	1a	Straight bar deadlift	5	6-8 reps	—	2-0-0	0.50-0.60
	1b	Band hamstring stretch	4	30 sec each side	2 min	—	—
	2a	One-arm dumbbell row	5	6-8 reps per side	—	2-0-0	0.40-0.50
	2b	Cat-camel stretch	4	10 reps	2 min	—	—
	3a	Barbell front squat	5	6-8 reps	—	2-0-0	0.50-0.60
	3b	Sumo stretch	4	30 sec	2 min	—	—
	4a	Loaded push-up	5	6-8 reps	—	2-0-0	0.40-0.50
	4b	Doorway pectoral stretch	4	30 sec	2 min	—	—

Core		EXERCISE	SETS	REPS, TIME	REST	TEMPO	VBT VELOCITY (M/SEC)
	1a	Plank	3	30 sec	—	—	—
	1b	Side plank	3	8 reps each side	1 min	—	—

Phase III: Mid–Off-Season

Submaximal and Maximal Strengths

Efficiency in any sport requires the ability to simultaneously recruit the primary muscles (prime movers) and fast-twitch muscle fibers as well as maintain the frequency of recruitment of those fibers. These traits rely primarily on having a sound foundation of maximal strength—the focus in phase III.

GOALS

- Promoting higher voluntary motor unit recruitment of the fast-twitch muscle fibers
- Increasing muscular endurance of short-to-medium durations
- Improving testosterone levels and relative strength

Submaximal Strength

TRAINING PARAMETERS

Training intensity	60%-80% 1RM
VBT velocity	0.50-0.75 m/sec (accelerative strength)
VBT velocity loss	20%-30%
Tempo	2-0-0
Reps	3-10
Sets	3-8
Rest	2-3 min
Frequency of training	3-4 times per week for upper- and lower-splits; 2-3 times per week for full body

SAMPLE PROGRAM

SAMPLE SUBMAXIMAL STRENGTH FULL-BODY PROGRAM

Warm-up		EXERCISE	SETS	TIME	REST	TEMPO	VBT VELOCITY (M/SEC)
	1	Tempo run	1	5 min	40 sec	—	—

Main (keep intensity between 60%-80% 1RM and velocity loss at 20%-30%)		EXERCISE	SETS	REPS, TIME	REST	TEMPO	VBT VELOCITY (M/SEC)
	1a	Romanian deadlift	5	5 reps	—	2-0-0	0.50-0.75
	1b	Prone hip rotator stretch	4	30 sec per side	2 min	—	—
	2a	Incline T-row	5	5 reps per side	—	2-0-0	0.45-0.55
	2b	Yoga plex	4	30 sec per side	2 min	—	—
	3a	Split squat	5	5 reps per side	—	2-0-0	0.50-0.75
	3b	Wall quad stretch	4	30 sec per side	2 min	—	—
	4a	Dumbbell bench press	5	5 reps	—	2-0-0	0.45-0.55
	4b	Sumo stretch	4	30 sec	2 min	—	—

Core		EXERCISE	SETS	REPS	REST	TEMPO	VBT VELOCITY (M/SEC)
	1a	Dead bug	3	8 per side	—	—	—
	1b	Half-kneeling cable chop	3	8 per side	—	—	—

Maximal Strength

TRAINING PARAMETERS

Training intensity	80%-95% 1RM
VBT velocity (concentric phase)	<0.50 m/sec
VBT velocity loss	20%-30%
Tempo	2-0-0
Reps	1-6
Sets	3-8
Rest	3-5 min
Frequency of training	3-4 times per week for upper- and lower-splits; 2-3 times per week for full body

SAMPLE PROGRAM

SAMPLE MAXIMAL STRENGTH FULL-BODY PROGRAM

Warm-up		EXERCISE	SETS	TIME	REST	TEMPO	VBT VELOCITY (M/SEC)
	1	Spin bike or Airdyne bike	1	5 min	—	—	—

Main (keep intensity between 80%-95% 1RM and velocity loss at 20%-30%)		EXERCISE	SETS	REPS, TIME	REST	TEMPO	VBT VELOCITY (M/SEC)
	1a	Straight-bar deadlift	5	3 reps	—	2-0-0	0.40-0.50
	1b	Hip CARS	4	5 reps per side	3 min	—	—
	2a	Barbell bench press	5	3 reps	—	2-0-0	0.35-0.45
	2b	Side-lying cross-body stretch	4	30 sec per side	3 min	—	—
	3a	Bilateral back squat	5	3 reps	—	2-0-0	0.40-0.50
	3b	Monster walk	4	5 reps per side	3 min	—	—
	4a	One-arm dumbbell row	5	3 reps per side	—	Explosive	0.35-0.45
	4b	Band lateral stretch	4	30 sec per side	3 min	—	—

Core		EXERCISE	SETS	REPS	REST	TEMPO	VBT VELOCITY (M/SEC)
	1a	Dead bug		8 per side	—	—	—
	1b	Half-kneeling cable chop	3	8 per side	—	—	—

Phase IV: Late Off-Season

Transfer to Sport-Specific Power

In Phase 4, we begin to take the strength adaptations developed in the previous phases and learn to apply them at faster rates. This is otherwise known as training "sport-specific power" and is crucial when competition nears.

GOALS

- Transferring strength gains into sport-specific power and muscular endurance
- Improving heart efficiency and lactate threshold
- Monitoring velocity or power loss to train explosive power and power endurance

Alactic Power

TRAINING PARAMETERS

Training Intensity	40%-80% 1RM (wherever peak power is achieved)
VBT velocity (concentric phase)	0.50-1.0 m/sec (wherever peak power is achieved)
VBT velocity or power loss	<10% 1RM
Tempo	Explosive
Reps	2-5 (<10 sec)
Sets	3-8
Rest	2-3 min
Frequency of training	2-3 times per week for full-body; 3-4 times per week for upper- and lower-splits

SAMPLE PROGRAM

SAMPLE ALACTIC POWER (STRENGTH-POWER) FULL-BODY PROGRAM FOR A HIGH SCHOOL OR COLLEGIATE BASEBALL ATHLETE

Warm-up		EXERCISE	SETS	TIME	REST	TEMPO	VBT VELOCITY (M/SEC)
	1	Tempo run	8	30 sec	1 min	—	—
Main (keep intensity between 40%-80% 1RM and velocity or power loss at <10%)		EXERCISE	SETS	REPS	REST	TEMPO	VBT VELOCITY (M/SEC)
	1a	Trap bar deadlift	6	5	2 min	Explosive	0.75-1.0
	2	Half-kneeling reverse cable row	6	5	2 min	Explosive	0.75-1.0
	3	Split squat	6	5 per side	2 min	Explosive	0.75-1.0
	4	Dumbbell bench-floor press	6	5	2 min	Explosive	0.60-0.80

Core		EXERCISE	SETS	REPS	REST	TEMPO	VBT VELOCITY (M/SEC)
	1a	Dead bug	2	8 per side	—	—	—
	1b	Half-kneeling cable chop	2	6 per side	—	—	—
	1c	Shoulder tap	2	10 per side	1 min	—	—
Conditioning		EXERCISE	SETS	DISTANCE	REST	TEMPO	VBT VELOCITY (M/SEC)
	1	Buildup	5	30 yd (27 m)	2 min	—	—

Lactic Power

TRAINING PARAMETERS

Intensity	20%-60% 1RM (wherever peak power is achieved)
VBT velocity	Lower body: 0.75-1.3 m/sec Upper body: 0.60-1.0 m/sec (strength-speed and speed-strength, wherever peak power is achieved)
VBT velocity loss	<10% 1RM
Tempo	Explosive
Reps	12-30
Sets	3-8
Rest	4-12 min
Frequency of training	2-3 times per week for full-body; 3-4 times per week for upper- and lower-splits

SAMPLE PROGRAM

SAMPLE LACTIC POWER (STRENGTH-POWER) FULL-BODY PROGRAM FOR A HIGH SCHOOL OR COLLEGIATE ICE HOCKEY ATHLETE

Warm-up		EXERCISE	SETS	TIME	REST	TEMPO	VBT VELOCITY (M/SEC)
	1	Tempo run	8	30 sec	1 min	—	—

Main (keep intensity between 20%-60% 1RM and velocity or power loss at <10%)		EXERCISE	SETS	REPS	REST	TEMPO	VBT VELOCITY (M/SEC)
	1	Trap bar deadlift	3	12	4 min	Explosive	Lower body: 0.75-1.3
	2	Prone seal row	3	15	3 min	Explosive	Upper body: 0.60-0.80
	3	Front squat	3	12	4 min	Explosive	Lower body: 0.75-1.3
	4	Dumbbell bench-floor press	3	15	3 min	Explosive	Upper body: 0.60-0.80

Core		EXERCISE	SETS	REPS	REST	TEMPO	VBT VELOCITY (M/SEC)
	1a	Dead bug	2	8 per side	—	—	—
	1b	Half-kneeling cable chop	2	6 per side	—	—	—
	1c	Shoulder tap	2	10 per side	1 min	—	—

Conditioning		EXERCISE	SETS	DISTANCE	REST	TEMPO	VBT VELOCITY (M/SEC)
	1	Buildup	5	30 yd (27 m)	2 min	—	—

Power Endurance (Capacity)

TRAINING PARAMETERS

Training intensity	20%-60% 1RM (wherever peak power is achieved)
VBT velocity (concentric phase)	0.75-1.3 m/sec (wherever peak power is achieved)
VBT velocity or power loss	<10%
Tempo	Explosive
Reps	Alactic power: 2-5 reps Lactic power: 12-30 reps
Series	2-4
Sets	3-6
Rest	5-20 sec between sets; 3-5 min between series
Frequency of training	2-3 times per week for full body; 3-4 times per week for upper- and lower-splits

SAMPLE PROGRAM

SAMPLE POWER ENDURANCE (SPEED-POWER) FULL-BODY PROGRAM FOR A HIGH SCHOOL OR COLLEGIATE FOOTBALL ATHLETE

Warm-up	EXERCISE	SETS	TIME	REST	TEMPO	VBT VELOCITY (M/SEC)
	1	Jump rope	1	5 min	—	—	—

Main (keep intensity between 20%-60% 1RM and velocity or power loss at <10%)		EXERCISE	SERIES	SETS × REPS	REST	TEMPO	VBT VELOCITY (M/SEC)
	1a	Power clean	2	5 × 5	2 min between sets; 4 min between series	Explosive	1.5-2.0 (peak velocity used on Olympic lifts)
	2	Trap bar jump (20%-40% of maximal strength)	2	5 × 3	20 sec between sets; 4 min between series	Explosive	1.0-1.3
	3	Kettlebell swing	2	5 × 5	20 sec between sets; 4 min between series	Explosive	1.0-1.3
	4	Barbell bench throw	2	5 × 3	20 sec between sets; 4 min between series	Explosive	0.85-1.0

Core		EXERCISE	SETS	REPS, BREATHS	REST	TEMPO	VBT VELOCITY (M/SEC)
	1a	Pallof press	2	8 reps per side	—	—	—
	1b	Wide-stance cable rotation	2	8 reps per side	—	—	—
	1c	Money maker	2	5 breaths	1 min	—	—

Conditioning		EXERCISE	SETS	TIME	REST	TEMPO	VBT VELOCITY (M/SEC)
	1	Sled sprint	5	8-10 sec	2 min	—	—

Muscular Endurance

TRAINING PARAMETERS

Training intensity	Short: 40%-60% 1RM
	Long: 20%-40% 1RM
VBT velocity (concentric phase)	Short: 0.60-1.0 m/sec
	Long: 0.85-1.3 m/sec
VBT velocity loss	Short: —
	Long: —
Tempo	Short: explosive
	Long: explosive
Reps	Short: 30 sec to 2 min per exercise
	Long: 2-8 min per exercise
Series	Short: 2-4
	Long: 2-4
Sets	Short: 2-6 sets per exercise
	Long: 1-3 sets per exercise
Rest	Short: 5-20 sec between sets; 3-5 min between series
	Long: 2-3 min between sets; 2-4 min between series

SAMPLE PROGRAMS

SAMPLE MUSCULAR ENDURANCE (SHORT, OR LACTIC CAPACITY) FULL-BODY PROGRAM FOR A HIGH SCHOOL OR COLLEGIATE SWIMMER (50-100 METER FLY)

Warm-up		EXERCISE	SETS	TIME	REST	TEMPO	VBT VELOCITY (M/SEC)
	1	Jump rope	3	2 min	1 min	—	—
Power plyometrics		EXERCISE	SETS	REPS	REST	TEMPO	VBT VELOCITY (M/SEC)
	1a	Sit-up to medicine ball overhead throw	2	5	—	Explosive	—
	1b	Box jump	2	5	1 min	Explosive	—
	2a	Sit-up to medicine ball chest pass	2	5	—	Explosive	—
	2b	Power step-up	2	5 per side	1 min	Explosive	—

Main (keep intensity between 40%-60% 1RM)		EXERCISE	SERIES	SETS × REPS OR TIME	REST	TEMPO	VBT VELOCITY (M/SEC)
	1	Split squat	2	4 × 30 sec	4 min between series; 15 sec between sets	Explosive	0.75-1.0
	2	Cable retraction to low row	2	4 × 30 sec	4 min between series; 15 sec between sets	—	0.60-0.70
	3	Band-resisted bench press	2	4 × 30 sec	4 min between series; 15 sec between sets	Explosive	0.60-0.70
	4	Triceps rope pull-down	2	4 × 30 sec	4 min between series; 15 sec between sets	Explosive	—
	5a	Half-kneeling cable lift	2	2 × 8 reps per side	30 sec	—	—
	5b	Side bridge	2	2 × 8 reps per side	1 min	—	—

Phase IV: Late Off-Season

SAMPLE MUSCULAR ENDURANCE (LONG, OR AEROBIC POWER) FULL-BODY PROGRAM FOR AN MMA ATHLETE

Warm-up		EXERCISE	SETS	TIME	REST	TEMPO	VBT VELOCITY (M/SEC)
	1	Jump rope	3	2 min	1 min	—	—

Power plyometrics		EXERCISE	SETS	REPS	REST	TEMPO	VBT VELOCITY (M/SEC)
	1a	Sit-up to medicine ball overhead throw	2	5	—	Explosive	—
	1b	Box jump	2	5	1 min	Explosive	—
	2a	Sit-up to medicine ball chest pass	2	5	—	Explosive	—
	2b	Power step-up	2	5 per side	1 min	Explosive	—

Main (keep intensity between 20%-40% 1RM)		EXERCISE	SERIES	SETS × TIME	REST	TEMPO	VBT VELOCITY (M/SEC)
	1	Bench hip bridge	2	2 × 120 sec	4 min between series; 10 sec between sets	Explosive	0.85-1.0
	2	Lat pull-down	2	2 × 120 sec	4 min between series; 10 sec between sets	Explosive	0.75-1.0
	3	Back squat	2	2 × 120 sec	4 min between series; 10 sec between sets	Explosive	0.85-1.0
	4	Band-resisted bench press	2	2 × 120 sec	4 min between series; 10 sec between sets	Explosive	0.75-1.0
	5	Seated dumbbell biceps curl	2	2 × 120 sec	4 min between series; 10 sec between sets	Explosive	—

Phase V: In-Season

Strength and Power Maintenance

Athletes in most sports need to maintain maximal strength, power, and power endurance (see table 11.2 on page 147 for strength proportion requirements for different sports during the season). Because in-season competition and practices limit training, these adaptations must all be trained together from week to week, from day to day, or sometimes even within the same day. All traits are important for optimizing performance; therefore, one should *not* take priority over another.

GOALS

- Managing training residuals
- Calculating specific strength proportions required for the sport

SAMPLE PROGRAM

SAMPLE TWO-DAY IN-SEASON FULL-BODY PROGRAM FOR A HIGH SCHOOL OR COLLEGIATE BASKETBALL PLAYER (MAXIMAL STRENGTH: 20 PERCENT; POWER: 60 PERCENT; POWER ENDURANCE: 20 PERCENT)

DAY 1						
Warm-up		EXERCISE	SETS	TIME	REST	TEMPO	VBT VELOCITY (M/SEC)
	1	Tempo run	8	30 sec	1 min	—	—
Main (keep intensity between 80%-90% 1RM and 20%-30% velocity loss for max strength, and intensity between 40%-60% 1RM and <10% velocity loss for power)		EXERCISE	SETS	REPS	REST	TEMPO	VBT VELOCITY (M/SEC)
	1	Max strength: back squat	3	3	3 min or as needed	2-0-0	0.40-0.50
	2	Max strength: barbell bench press	3	3	3 min or as needed	2-0-0	0.35-0.45
	3	Power: trap bar deadlift	4	4	2 min	Explosive	0.75-1.0
	4	Power: bilateral cable row	4	4	2 min	Explosive	0.60-0.70
	5	Power: lateral dumbbell lunge	4	4	2 min	Explosive	0.75-1.0
Core	1a	Dead bug	2	6 per side	—	—	—
	1b	Pallof press with hold	2	6 per side	1 min	0-5-0	—

DAY 2						
Warm-up	**EXERCISE**	**SETS**	**REPS, TIME**	**REST**	**TEMPO**	**VBT VELOCITY (M/SEC)**
	1 Mobility circuit	1	—	—	—	—
Main (keep intensity between 20%-60% 1RM for power endurance and 40%-60% 1RM for power, and power losses at <10%)	**EXERCISE**	**SERIES**	**SETS × REPS**	**REST**	**TEMPO**	**VBT VELOCITY (M/SEC)**
	1 Power: trap bar jump	2	6 × 3	10 sec between sets; 3 min between series	Explosive	1.8-2.0 (use peak velocities)
	2 Power: barbell bench throw	2	6 × 3	10 sec between sets; 3 min between series	Explosive	1.8-2.0 (use peak velocities)
	EXERCISE	**SETS**	**REPS**	**REST**	**TEMPO**	**VBT VELOCITY (M/SEC)**
	3 Power endurance: back squat	4	4	3 min	Explosive	0.75-1.0
	4 Power endurance: band-assisted push-up	4	4	3 min	Explosive	0.60-0.70
	5 Power endurance: split squat	4	4	3 min	Explosive	0.75-1.0
Core	**EXERCISE**	**SETS**	**REPS**	**REST**	**TEMPO**	**VBT VELOCITY (M/SEC)**
	1a Dead bug	2	8 per side	—	—	—
	1b Half-kneeling cable chop	2	8 per side	—	—	—

Program periodization is an art unto itself. There are many great books on the topic, and I recommend that you purchase a few and begin taking that journey in order to help you better implement VBT. It is also important to understand that, while using VBT to prescribe loads and monitor fatigue can be a game changer for making strength and speed gains, what is appropriate for one athlete may not be appropriate for another. Taking into account variables such as height, weight, training age, and fiber density can put two athletes at opposite ends of a strength zone. The only true way to program efficiently is to create profiles for each athlete and use autoregulation daily to monitor fatigue. This will give both the coach and the athlete the best opportunity for success in the weight room and on the field.

Bibliography

Introduction

Mann, J.B. 2016. *Developing Explosive Athletes: Use of Velocity-Based Training in Training Athletes*. 1st ed. Self-published, CreateSpace.

Chapter 1

Flanagan, E.P., and M. Jovanovic. 2014. "Researched Applications of Velocity Based Strength Training." *Journal of Australian Strength & Conditioning* 22:58-69. www.researchgate.net/publication/265227430_Researched_Applications_of_Velocity_Based_Streng.

González-Badillo, J.J, and L. Sánchez-Medina. 2010. "Movement Velocity as a Measure of Loading Intensity in Resistance Training." *International Journal of Sports Medicine* 31(5):347-352. www.ncbi.nlm.nih.gov/pubmed/20180176.

Jidovtseff, B., Harris, N.K., Crielaard, J.M., and J.B. Cronin. 2011. "Using the Load–Velocity Relationship for 1RM Prediction. *Journal of Strength and Conditioning Research* 25(1):267-270. www.ncbi.nlm.nih.gov/pubmed/19966589.

Loturco, I., Kobal, R., Morales, J.E., Kitamura, K., Cal Abad, C.C., Pereira, L.A., and F.Y. Nakamura. 2017. "Predicting the Maximum Dynamic Strength in Bench Press: The High Precision of the Bar Velocity Approach. *Journal of Strength and Conditioning Research* 31(4):1127-1131.

Mann, J.B., Thyfault, J.P., Ivey, P.A., and S.P. Sayers. 2010. "The Effect of Autoregulatory Progressive Resistance Exercise vs. Linear Periodization on Strength Improvement in College Athletes." *Journal of Strength and Conditioning Research* 24(7):1718-23. www.ncbi.nlm.nih.gov/pubmed/20543732.

Mann, J.B. 2016. *Developing Explosive Athletes: Use of Velocity-Based Training in Training Athletes*. 1st ed. Self-published, CreateSpace.

NCAA. n.d. "Velocity Based Training." Health and Safety. Accessed May 9, 2017. www.ncaa.org/health-and-safety/sport-science-institute/velocity-based-training.

Ormsbee M.J., Carzoli, J., Klemp, A., Allman, B., Zourdos, M.C., Jeong-Su, K., and L. Panton. 2017. "Efficacy of the Repetitions in Reserve-Based Rating of Perceived Exertion for the Bench Press in Experienced and Novice Benchers. *Journal of Strength and Conditioning Research* 33(2):337-345. www.researchgate.net/publication/315195335_Efficacy_Of_The_Repetitions_In_Reserve-Based_Rating_Of_Perceived_Exertion_For_The_Bench_Press_In_Experienced_And_Novice_Benchers.

Plofker, C. n.d. "Velocity-Based Training Options for Strength." *Simplifaster* (blog). Accessed November 10, 2020. https://simplifaster.com/articles/velocity-based-training-options-strength/

Randell, A.D., Cronin, J.B., Keogh, J.W.L., Gill, N.D., and M.C. Pedersen. 2011. "Effect of Instantaneous Performance Feedback During 6 Weeks of Velocity-Based Resistance Training on Sport-Specific Performance Tests. *Journal of Strength and Conditioning Research* 25(1):87-93. www.ncbi.nlm.nih.gov/pubmed/21157389.

Science for Sport. "Velocity Based Training." Velocity Based Training. Last modified August 5, 2017. www.scienceforsport.com/velocity-based-training/.

Wulf, G. 2012. "Attentional Focus and Motor Learning: A Review of 15 Years. *International Review of Sport and Exercise Physiology* 6(1):77-104. https://doi.org/10.1080/1750984X.2012.723728.

Chapter 2

Baker, D. 2014. "An Intro to Velocity Based Training." *Push* (blog), *Train with Push*. February 14, 2014.

www.trainwithpush.com/blog/an-intro-to-velocity-based-training.

Crewther, B., Cronin, J., and J. Keogh. 2006. "Possible Stimuli for Strength and Power Adaptation: Acute Metabolic Responses. *Sports medicine (Auckland, N.Z.)* 36:65-78.

González-Badillo, J.J., and L. Sánchez-Medina. 2010. "Movement Velocity as a Measure of Loading Intensity in Resistance Training." *International Journal of Sports Medicine* 31:347-352.

González-Badillo, J.J., Marques, M.C., and L. Sánchez-Medina. 2011. "The Importance of Movement Velocity as a Measure to Control Resistance Training Intensity." *Journal of Human Kinetics* 29A:15-19.

Kraemer, W.J., and N.A. Ratamess. 2004. "Fundamentals of Resistance Training: Progression and Exercise Prescription." *Medicine & Science in Sports & Exercise* 36(4):674-688. https://doi.org/10.1249/01.mss.0000121945.36635.61.

Loturco, I., Nakamura, F.Y., Tricoli, V., Kobal, R., Abad, C.C.C., Kitamura, K., Ugrinowitsch, C., Gil, S., Pereira, L.A., and J.J. González-Badillo. 2015. "Determining the Optimum Power Load in Jump Squat Using the Mean Propulsive Velocity. *PLoS ONE* 10:(10):e0140102. https://doi.org/10.1371/journal.pone.0140102.

Sánchez-Medina, L., Perez, C.E., and J.J. González-Badillo. 2010. "Importance of the Propulsive Phase in Strength Assessment." *International Journal of Sports Medicine* 31:123-129. https://doi.org/10.1055/s-0029-1242815.

Walker, O. 2017. "Velocity Based Training." 2017. *Science for Sport* (blog). August 5, 2017. www.scienceforsport.com/velocity-based-training.

Chapter 3

Cronin, J.B., Hing, R.D., and P.J. McNair. 2004. "Reliability and Validity of a Linear Position Transducer for Measuring Jump Performance." *The Journal of Strength and Conditioning Research* 18(3):590-593. https://doi.org/10.1519/00124278-200408000-00035.

Donnelly, S. n.d. "Get Started With Your PUSH Band." Getting Started. Accessed November 5, 2020. https://intercom.help/pushcenter/en/articles/2865620-get-started-with-your-push-band.

Hansen, K.T., Cronin, J.B., and M.J. Newton. 2011. "The Reliability of Linear Position Transducer, Force Plate and Combined Measurement of Explosive Power-Time Variables During a Loaded Jump Squat in Elite Athletes." *Sports Biomechanics* 10(1):46-58. https://doi.org/10.1080/14763141.2010.547592.

Pareja-Blanco F., Rodríguez-Rosell, D., Sánchez-Medina, L., Sanchis-Moysi, J., Dorado, C., Mora-Custodio, R., Yáñez-García, J.M., et al. 2016. "Effects of Velocity Loss During Resistance Training on Athletic Performance, Strength Gains and Muscle Adaptations." *Scandinavian Journal of Medicine & Science in Sports* 27(7):724-735. https://doi.org/doi:10.1111/sms.12678.

Valle, C. n.d. "Getting Started with Velocity-Based Training and GymAware." *SimpliFaster* (blog). Accessed November 10, 2020. https://simplifaster.com/articles/velocity-based-training-gymaware/.

Chapter 4

Bowhay, S. 2020. "Implementing VBT in Professional Soccer." Filmed April 20, 2020. 1:13:13. www.youtube.com/watch?v=938n3hTEjng.

Mann, J.B. 2016. *Developing Explosive Athletes: Use of Velocity Based Training in Athletes.* 1st ed. Self-published, CreateSpace.

Sevin, T. n.d. "Strength Continuum in Resistance Training: Answering the 'Why.'" *SimpliFaster* (blog). Accessed November 10, 2020. https://simplifaster.com/articles/resistance-training-strength-continuum.

Valle, C. n.d. "Force-Velocity Profiling and Prescription With Athletes." *SimpliFaster* (blog). Accessed November 10, 2020. https://simplifaster.com/articles/force-velocity-profiling.

Chapter 5

González-Badillo, J.J., and L. Sánchez-Medina. 2010. "Movement Velocity as a Measure of Loading Intensity in Resistance Training." *International Journal of Sports Medicine* 31:347-352.

Jidovtseff B., Quièvre J., Hanon C., and J.M. Crielaard. 2009 "Inertial Muscle Profiles Allow a More Accurate Training Loads Definition." *Sport & Science* 24(2), 91-96.

Izquierdo, M., González-Badillo, J.J., Häkkinen, K., Ibañez, J., Kraemer, W.J., Altadill, A., Eslava, J., and E.M. Gorostiaga. 2006. "Effect of Loading on Unintentional Lifting Velocity Declines During Single Sets of Repetitions to Failure During Upper and Lower Extremity Muscle Actions." *International Journal of Sports Medicine* 27:718-724. www.ncbi.nlm.nih.gov/pubmed/16944400.

Mann, J.B. 2016. *Developing Explosive Athletes: Use of Velocity-Based Training in Training Athletes.* 1st ed. Self-published, CreateSpace.

Science for Sport. "Velocity Based Training." Velocity Based Training. Last modified August 5, 2017. www.scienceforsport.com/velocity-based-training/.

Chapter 6

Baker, D. 2018. "Fatigue From Other Training and Its Effects Upon Velocity Scores." *Dan Baker Strength* (blog). January 16, 2018. www.danbakerstrength.com/blog/2018/1/16/fatigue-from-other-training-and-its-effects-upon-velocity-scores

Brooks, G.A., Fahey, T.D., and K.M. Baldwin. 2004. *Exercise Physiology: Human Bioenergetics and Its Applications, Fourth Edition.* New York, NY: McGraw-Hill Education.

Davis, J.M., and S.P. Bailey. 1997. "Possible Mechanisms of Central Nervous System Fatigue During Exercise." *Medicine & Science in Sports & Exercise* 29:45-57.

Flanagan, E.P., and M. Jovanovic. 2014. "Researched Applications of Velocity Based Strength Training." *Journal of Australian Strength & Conditioning* 22:58-69. www.researchgate.net/publication/265227430_Researched_Applications_of_Velocity_Based_Streng.

Folland, J.P., Irish, C.S., Roberts, J.C., Tarr, J.E., and D.A. Jones. 2002. "Fatigue Is not a Necessary Stimulus for Strength Gains During Resistance Training." *British Journal of Sports Medicine* 36: 370-74.

Francis, C. 2012. *The Charlie Francis Training System*. Amazon Digital Services, LLC. Kindle.

Gambetta, V. n.d. "Defining Supercompensation Training." *Human Kinetics* (blog). Accessed November 10, 2020.

https://us.humankinetics.com/blogs/excerpt/defining-supercompensation-training.

Jidovtseff, B., Harris, N.K., Crielaard, J.M., and J.B. Cronin. 2011. "Using the Load–Velocity Relationship for 1RM Prediction." *Journal of Strength and Conditioning Research* 25(1):267-270.

Juggernaut Training Systems. 2019. "The JuggLife | Velocity Based Training | Dr. Bryan Mann." Filmed October 29, 2019. 41:05. www.youtube.com/watch?v=i1cPTBQn_Vw.

Mann, J.B. 2016. *Developing Explosive Athletes: Use of Velocity Based Training in Athletes*. 1st ed. Self-published, CreateSpace.

Mann, J.B., Thyfault, J.P., Ivey, P.A., and S.P. Sayers. 2010. "The Effect of Autoregulatory Progressive Resistance Exercise vs. Linear Periodization on Strength Improvement in College Athletes." *Journal of Strength and Conditioning Research* 24:1718-1723. www.ncbi.nlm.nih.gov/pubmed/20543732.

Nevin, J, 2019. "Autoregulated Resistance Training: Does Velocity-Based Training Represent the Future?" *Strength and Conditioning Journal* 41:34-39. https://doi.org/10.1519/SSC.0000000000000471

Pareja-Blanco, F., Alcazar, J., Sánchez-Valdepeñas, Cornejo-Daza, P.J., Piqueras-Sanchiz, F., Mora-Vela, R., Sánchez-Moreno, M., Bachero-Mena, B., Ortega-Becerra, M., and L.M. Alegre. 2020. "Velocity Loss as a Critical Variable Determining the Adaptations to Strength Training." *Medicine & Science in Sports & Exercise* 52:1752-1762. https://doi.org/10.1249/MSS.0000000000002295.

Pareja-Blanco, F., Rodríguez-Rosell, D., Sánchez-Medina, L., Sanchis-Moysi, J., Dorado, C., Mora-Custodio, R., Yáñez-García, J.M., et al. 2016 "Effects of Velocity Loss During Resistance Training on Athletic Performance, Strength Gains and Muscle Adaptations." *Scandinavian Journal of Medicine & Science in Sports* 27:724-735.

Sánchez-Medina, L., and J.J. González-Badillo. 2011. "Velocity Loss as an Indicator of Neuromuscular Fatigue During Resistance Training." *Medicine & Science in Sports & Exercise* 43:1725-1734. https://doi.org/10.1249/MSS.0b013e318213f880.

Selye, H. 1956. *The Stress of Life*. New York: McGraw-Hill Book Company, Inc.

Verkoshansky, Y.V. 1989. *Fundamentals of Special Strength Training in Sports*. Livonia, Michigan: Sportivny Press.

Chapter 7

Bompa, T., and Buzzichelli, C. 2015. *Periodization Training for Sports*. 3rd ed. Champaign, IL: Human Kinetics.

Haff, G., and N. Triplett, eds. 2016. *Essentials of Strength Training and Conditioning, Fourth Edition*. Champaign, IL: Human Kinetics.

Haff, G., and E. Haff. 2012. "Training Integration and Periodization." In *NSCA's Guide to Program Design*, edited by J. Hoffman, 209-254. Champaign, IL: Human Kinetics.

Perch. n.d. "Periodization and Programming With VBT." *Perch* (blog). Accessed November 10, 2020. www.perch.fit/blog/periodization-and-programming-with-vbt/.

Poliquin, C. 1988. "Five Steps to Increasing the Effectiveness of Your Strength Training Program". *National Strength and Conditioning Association Journal* 10:34-39.

Signore, N. April, 2018. "A Guide to Training Strength and Power With Velocity-Based Training." Webinar.

Chapter 8

Bompa, T., and Buzzichelli, C. 2015. *Periodization Training for Sports*. 3rd ed. Champaign, IL: Human Kinetics.

Bondarchuk, A.P. 2014. *The Olympian Manual for Strength & Size: Blue Print From the World's Greatest Coach*. Muskegon, MI: Ultimate Athlete Concepts.

Haff, G., and N. Triplett, eds. 2016. *Essentials of Strength Training and Conditioning, Fourth Edition*. Champaign, IL: Human Kinetics.

Signore, N. April 2018. "A Guide to Training Strength and Power With Velocity-Based Training." Webinar.

Knobloch K. 2007. "Eccentric Rehabilitation Exercise Increases Peritendinous Type I Collagen Synthesis in Humans With Achilles Tendinosis." *Scandinavian Journal Of Medicine & Science in Sports*, *17*(3), 298–299. https://doi.org/10.1111/j.1600-0838.2007.00652.x

Chapter 9

Bompa, T., and Buzzichelli, C. 2015. *Periodization Training for Sports*. 3rd ed. Champaign, IL: Human Kinetics.

Haff, G., and N. Triplett, eds. 2016. *Essentials of Strength Training and Conditioning, Fourth Edition*. Champaign, IL: Human Kinetics.

Howard, J.D., Ritchie, M.R., Gater, D.A., Gater, D.R., and R.M. Enoka. 1985. "Determining Factors of Strength: Physiological Foundations." *National Strength and Conditioning Journal* 7:16-21.

Signore, N. "A Guide to Training Strength and Power With Velocity-Based Training." Webinar.

Chapter 10

Bompa, T., and Buzzichelli, C. 2015. *Periodization Training for Sports*. 3rd ed. Champaign, IL: Human Kinetics.

Bondarchuk, A.P. 2014 *The Olympian Manual for Strength & Size: Blue Print From the World's Greatest Coach*. Muskegon, MI: Ultimate Athlete Concepts.

Haff, G., and N. Triplett, eds. 2016. *Essentials of Strength Training and Conditioning, Fourth Edition*. Champaign, IL: Human Kinetics.

Mann, J.B. 2016. *Developing Explosive Athletes: Use of Velocity-Based Training in Training Athletes*. 1st ed. Self-published, CreateSpace.

Pareja-Blanco F., Rodríguez-Rosell, D., Sánchez-Medina, L., Sanchis-Moysi, J., Dorado, C., Mora-Custodio, R., Yáñez-García, J.M., et al. 2016. "Effects of Velocity Loss During Resistance Training on Athletic Performance, Strength Gains and Muscle Adaptations." *Scandinavian Journal of Medicine & Science in Sports* 27(7):724-735. https://doi.org/doi:10.1111/sms.12678.

Signore, N. April, 2018. "A Guide to Training Strength and Power With Velocity-Based Training." Webinar.

Simmons, L. 2007. *The Westside Barbell Book of Methods*. Columbus, OH: Westside Barbell.

Chapter 11

Bompa, T., and Buzzichelli, C. 2015. *Periodization Training for Sports.* 3rd ed. Champaign, IL: Human Kinetics.

Haff, G., and Triplett, N., eds. 2016. *Essentials of Strength Training and Conditioning.* 4th ed. Champaign, IL: Human Kinetics.

Issurin, V. 2008. *Block Periodization: Breakthrough in Sport Training.* Muskegon, MI: Ultimate Athlete Concepts.

Winkelman, N. 2012. "Athlete Profiling: Choosing a Periodization System to Maximize Individual Performance." Filmed July 11-14, 2012. 1:10:17. www.youtube.com/watch?v=jIGebkccLkc.

Index

A

absolute strength zone 46-47. *See also* maximal strength training

accelerative strength zone 48-49. *See also* submaximal strength training

accelerometers

    basic setup 33-36

    data interpretation 36-39

    described 29-30

    factors in choosing 39

    for 1RM testing 62

    pros and cons 30

accountability, in athletes 9, 11

adaptation

    detraining and training residuals 143, 144-146, 150

    special strength zones and 43-45, 58

    sport-specific 130-132

    velocity loss monitoring and 73-80

aerobic capacity 139

aerobic power 139

alactic power

    described 128, 130

    fatigue and 130

    sample full-body programs 133-134, 161-162

    training parameters 133, 161

athlete readiness

    stress and 12-13, 70

    testing for 80, 81-83

    velocity monitoring and 70-73

autoregulation

    described 12, 70

    VBT data and 37-38, 72-73

    velocity loss and 83

B

ballistic exercises

    defined 22

    in power endurance training 137

    in transition I phase 131-132

Bar Sensei. *See* accelerometers

baseball sample programs

    alactic power 161-162

    yearly training plan 86, 93

basketball sample maintenance programs 149-150, 168-169

body weight 64-65

Bompa, Tudor 146-147

C

central nervous system (CNS) 69

CNS fatigue 69-70, 81-83

competitiveness 9-10

competitive period (in-season)

    adaptation decline in 143

    described 93

    focus and exercises in 96

    goals for 144-147

    sample programs 149-150, 168-169

concentric contraction 17-19

D

deceleration 19

detraining

    avoiding 150

    contributing factors 146

    programming and 143-144

    training residuals 145

E

early off-season

    considerations in 101

    described 93

    focus and exercises in 94

    hypertrophy phases 106-114, 155-157

    tissue prep phase 102-105, 153-154

eccentric contractions 16-17

endurance sports 128-129, 146

energy systems

    muscular endurance and 139

    power types and 128, 130

exercises

    absolute strength zone 47

About the Author

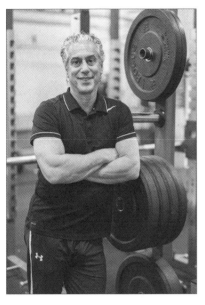

Nunzio Signore is a certified strength and conditioning coach and the owner and operator of Rockland Peak Performance (RPP). He is also a member of the American Baseball Biomechanics Society (ABBS) and director of the Pitching Lab in New Jersey. For the past 10 years, he has been one of the most in-demand strength and conditioning coaches in the New York and New Jersey areas, working with players from the Minnesota Twins, Anaheim Angels, New York Yankees, New York Mets, Arizona Diamondbacks, and Seattle Mariners, to name a few. He has written articles for publications such as *Inside Pitch Magazine* and speaks annually at baseball clinics such as Pitch-a-Palooza, Bridge the Gap, NY Coaches Convention, Be the Best, and Inside Baseball Coaches Conventions.

Signore also has served as an adjunct professor at St. Thomas Aquinas College, teaching theories and applications of strength and conditioning. In addition, he is a lecturer at Springfield College, SUNY Cortland, and Penn State and is affiliated with the Wake Forest Pitching Lab.

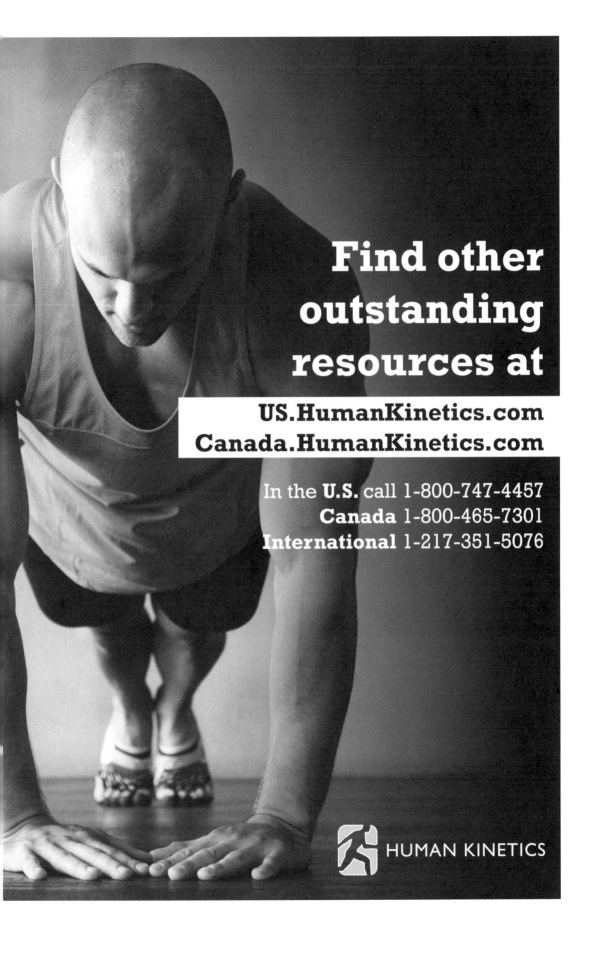